Network Policy Making within the Turkish Health Sector

Network Policy Making within the Turkish Health Sector: Becoming Collaborative

BY

JULINDA HOXHA
Bilkent University, Turkey

emerald
PUBLISHING

United Kingdom – North America – Japan – India – Malaysia – China

Emerald Publishing Limited
Howard House, Wagon Lane, Bingley BD16 1WA, UK

First edition 2020

Reprints and permissions service
Contact: permissions@emeraldinsight.com

British Library Cataloguing in Publication Data
A catalogue record for this book is available from the British Library

ISBN: 978-1-83867-095-5 (Print)
ISBN: 978-1-83867-094-8 (Online)
ISBN: 978-1-83867-096-2 (Epub)

Printed and bound by CPI Group (UK) Ltd, Croydon, CR0 4YY

ISOQAR certified Management System, awarded to Emerald for adherence to Environmental standard ISO 14001:2004.

ISOQAR REGISTERED
Certificate Number 1985
ISO 14001

INVESTOR IN PEOPLE

Contents

List of Tables and Figures

List of Terms and Abbreviations

AKP	Justice and Development Party (Adalet ve Kalkınma Partisi)
ATO	Ankara Chamber of Commerce (Ankara Ticaret Odası)
BLT Model	Build Lease Transfer Model
CHP	Republican People's Party (Cumhuriyet Halk Partisi)
CMHC	Community Mental Health Centers
ÇPSSGP	Program for Improving Multi-Sectoral Health Responsibility (Çok Paydaşlı Sağlık Sorumluluğunu Geliştirme Proğramı)
DEİK	Foreign Economic Relations Board (Dış Ekonomik İlişkiler Kurulu)
EU	European Union
EVSAD	Home Healthcare and Social Services Association (Evde Sağlık ve Sosyal Hizmetler Derneği)
GDP	Gross Domestic Product
GNA	Turkısh Grand National Assembly
HTA	Health Technology Assessment
HTP	Health Transformation Programme
IT	Information Technology
MHSA	Ministry of Health and Social Affairs
MoFSP	Ministry of Family and Social Policies
MoH	Ministry of Health
NCC	Network Collaborative Capacity
NGO	Non-Governmental Organization
NGS	Network Governance School
NHIS	National Health Information System
OECD	Organization for Economic Cooperation and Development
PPP	Public–Private Partnership
RDA	Regional Development Agencies
SATURK	Health Tourism Coordination Council (Sağlık Turizmi Koordinasyon Kurulu)
SHÇEK	Social Services and Child Protection Agency (Sosyal Hizmetler ve Çocuk Esirgeme Kurumu)
SME	Small and Medium Size Enterprises

SPO	State Planning Organization
SRDC	Software Research and Development Consultancy Limited
SSI	Social Security Institution
SYDV	Social Assistance and Solidarity Foundations (Sosyal Yardımlaşma ve Dayanışma Vakfı)
TAPDK	Tobacco and Alcohol Market Regulatory Authority (Tütün ve Alkol Piyasası Düzenleme Kurumu)
TİKA	Turkish Cooperation and Coordination Agency (Türk İşbirliği ve Koordinasyon Başkanlığı)
TMMDA	Turkish Medicines and Medical Devices Agency
TMMOB	Turkish Chamber of Engineers and Architects (Türk Mühendis ve Mimar Odaları Birliği)
TOBB	The Union of Chamber and Commodity Exchanges of Turkey (Türkiye Odalar ve Borsalar Birliği)
TÜİK	Turkish Statistical Institute (Türkiye İstatistik Kurumu)
WB	World Bank
WHO	World Health Organization
YÖK	The Council of Higher Education (Yüksek Öğretim Kurulu)

Acknowledgments

> To understand matters rightly we should understand their details; and as that knowledge is almost infinite, our knowledge is always superficial and imperfect.(La Rouchefoucauld, *The Maxims*, 1678)

We owe so much to those people, who sometimes through their help and motivation but even more so through their critique keep us moving forward in our knowledge seeking endeavors. Here, I can only mention but a few who had a direct influence on my work. First of all, I am deeply indebted to Professor Metin Heper for his unrelenting support and guidance throughout the whole process of book writing. I am also very grateful to Associate Professor Saime Özçürümez, who encouraged me to explore some of the most relevant and salient research puzzles within the field of comparative politics and convinced me of the need to do research on the topic of this book. I would also like to thank Professor Mete Yıldız, Associate Professor Zeynep Kadirbeyoğlu, and Associate Professor Çağla Ökten, who have been very helpful in highlighting some of the main limitations as well as possibilities for improvement in my research through their constructive criticism. My special thanks go to Associate Professor Anne Mette Kjær for her readiness to help while preparing the book proposal. I am also very thankful to Eliza Gheorghe, Christina Hamer, Jermaine Ma, Amanda Hayes, and Petra Cafnik Uludağ for all their comments and suggestions throughout the process of book writing. Last but not least, I deeply thank my parents Ylli and Bukurije, my husband Saimir, and my children Emin and Sara. They are the motivation that makes me work harder each day. My biggest hope is to be their source of motivation one day in the future.

Foreword

Little is known about network policy making in less advanced democracies. This is particularly the case in low- and middle-income countries. In the latter countries, little effort has been made to come up with systematic and cross-national studies of policy networks. In the process, the networks in such places have generally remained only as metaphors and "theoretical" perspectives.

Turkey is a middle-income country. Despite its "structural and cultural constrains" the country has made an effort to join the club of developed economies, basically through adopting the latter's policy models. This has been the case particularly in the health sector, public health, health tourism, and the medical industry.

The present book examines the conditions under which said policy networks have emerged and thrived in Turkey by, not unexpectedly, drawing upon the health policy sector. While recent policy studies in Turkey have employed macro-level institutional analysis, this book has adopted a micro–meso level analysis of policy processes, focusing on the investigation of the (policy) networks within the health policy sub-areas.

As the present author has pointed out elsewhere (Heper, 1993), in Turkey while both societal and political elites have been expected to play an active role toward policy making in the name of "general interest," studies on the Turkish case have shown that societal actors have traditionally had minimal or no impact on public policy making due to the impediments such as populism, clientelism, and opportunities (Heper & Yıldırım, 2011).

More recently, the networks in Turkey have turned out to be the effective channels of societal participation. Lately, the expert involvement in the said policy making processes and the tools that provide legitimacy to those processes, have been at the heart of public policy issues.

In her book, Julinda Hoxha has skillfully traced the past and present odyssey in question.

In essence, in solitude.

Prof. Dr. Metin Heper
Bilkent University

References

Heper, M. (1993). Political culture as a dimension of compatibility. In M. Heper, A. Öncü, & H. Kramer (Eds.), *Turkey and the west: Changing political and cultural identities* (pp. 16–17). London: IB Tauris.

Heper, M., & Yıldırım, S. (2011). Revisiting civil society in Turkey. *Journal of Southeast European and Black Sea Studies*, *11*(1), 1–18.

Chapter 1

Introduction: Extending the Study of Policy Networks Beyond Their Original Context

Abstract

This book is aimed at extending the study of network collaboration beyond the context of advanced democracies through the exploration of policy networks in Turkey – a country with statist policy style and authoritarian political culture. The focus here will be on cross-sectoral collaboration taking place within the Turkish health sector – a policy area that has been steadily improving with the initiation of the Health Transformation Programme (HTP) in 2003. To date, many scholars have studied the outcomes of the HTP reforms on the healthcare system including indicators such as healthcare access, health insurance coverage and healthcare services. However, despite the transformative nature of the program, a limited number of studies have assessed the impact of HTP reforms on changing policy and governance patterns in Turkey. Considering this gap in the literature, the aim of this book is to empirically examine the context, capacity and consequences of cross-sectoral collaboration within the health sector in Turkey through a micro- and meso-level investigation of policy networks developed in the sub-areas of public health, medical industry, and health tourism covering the years between 2011 and 2015. Furthermore, this book provides an account of those factors that impede cross-sectoral arrangements from turning into venues of policy collaboration. Such juxtaposition is designed to enhance the understanding of policy networks as conceptual devices and practical tools of collaboration in public policy.

Keywords: Authoritarianism; expert interviews; governance; middle-range theory; policy networks; Turkey

Network Policy Making within the Turkish Health Sector: Becoming Collaborative, 1–16

doi:10.1108/978-1-83867-094-820201002

Unpacking Networks: Redundant Conceptual Devices or Practical Policy Instruments?

When I commenced writing this book, I contemplated the renowned work of Theodore J. Lowi, whose legacy continues to guide contemporary debates and scholarly research in the fields of political science and public administration to this day:

> [...] prevailing fashions in political science have put heaviest stress on the politics rather than the government side of the field. In many dimensions of politics there are well-developed vocabularies, indicating indeed where the major theoretical interests have been. Students of politics do occasionally turn to policy and government, but the tendency has been to do so only because the interesting conflicts are around issues, and many issues involve basic policies. But the issue of policy was not the part of these issues that came in for serious analysis. (Lowi, 1972, p. 299)

Two issues are being emphasized in this paragraph with insights on the interplay of policy and politics. First, over the years politics has been overestimated at the expense of policy. Secondly, policy is perceived as a function of politics under the commonly known expression that "politics determines policies." As a result, policy has remained in the shadow of politics, especially in those countries where authoritarian politics is considered to be omnipresent through its impact on all spheres of society from the state apparatus to individual lifestyles. The link between politics and policy is undeniable. Hall and Jenkins (2003) argue that "[p]ublic policy cannot remain independent of the political process and cannot be value free" (p. 3). However, the mission of this book is to expand the policy horizons beyond the confines of political orientations, by bringing policy to the attention of policy makers, policy practitioners, researchers, and students as a separate sphere of influence that can change the lives of individual citizens independent of political pressures and incentives. Policy processes and outcomes might be less noticeable, yet, they turn out to be more durable compared to abrupt political, economic, and social transformations. Pierson (2000) maintains that policy effects are accumulated over time in a steady fashion and turn out to be "remarkably durable" especially when they are "grounded in law" (p. 259).

Following this logic, policy analysis has focused its attention toward legal decision-making in policy processes and the formation of the *policy regimes* as relatively stable institutional arrangements. According to Sabel and Simon (2012), policy regimes "engage a diverse variety of participants" including coalitions of public, private, and voluntary actors and "do not have the top-down, command-and-control structure" observed in government regulations (p. 1267). Moreover, "neither do they arise spontaneously" which contributes to their relatively long-term nature (Sabel & Simon, 2012, p. 1267). According to this definition, policy regimes are influenced by politics; but, they are less prone to politicization. Therefore, they constitute a relatively autonomous sphere of policy making. Acknowledging their importance, scholars focus on the role of exogenous shocks leading to the formation of these regimes, political coalitions that contribute to their preservation, or the effectiveness of these regimes through macro-level policy analysis.

Conversely, less attention has been paid to the operational side of the policy making within these regimes or the ostensible practice of policy making through micro- and meso-level policy analysis. The practice of policy making includes daily activities and relations among actors at different levels of governance which represent what Freeman, Griggs, and Boaz (2011) identify as the "often unexplored elements of policy" (p. 131). In an attempt to tackle different policy related problems, policy practice may naturally result in cooperation, competition, and even conflict among actors. In the presence of all possible outcomes, the practice of policy making that takes place among professionals within and outside the government is inherently less prone to conflict compared to debates that take place in political arenas. Laws and Hajer (2006) affirm that eventually the policy practice is more conducive to cooperative tendencies among involved actors who are willing to overcome policy challenges in a collaborative fashion through tools of policy innovation and improvisation.

These cooperative tendencies within the practice of policy making can be studied through the lenses of the network approach which has become increasingly popular, attracting significant attention among scholars in the fields of political science and public administration. *Networks* entered the political vocabulary in the 1980s and played a central role among scholars ever since. Networks were initially considered to be ground-breaking phenomena due to their primary concern with the involvement of non-state actors in policy making processes. Mayntz (1993) explains that they manifested as "partly autonomous societal subsystems ... that enjoy some degree of autonomy" (p. 2), which seemed to bring the glory of impartial and non-politicized policy making back to the scholarly agenda. Some scholars have argued that policy networks constitute a substantial break from the traditional governing mechanisms and represent a new pattern of governance besides hierarchical bureaucracies and competitive markets (Rhodes, 1996, 1997, 2007; Sørensen, 2002, 2005, 2006; Sørensen & Torfing, 2005, 2007, 2009, 2016; Stoker, 1998, 2006). Due to their growing significance, many governance-related phenomena have been revisited and redefined considering the network concept to the extent that policy networks have often been perceived as equivalent to the concept of governance itself. Following this logic, Stoker (1998) argues that governance is ultimately "about autonomous self-governing networks of actors" (p. 23). As a result, a massive collection of literature exists which examines policy networks as a discrete mode of governance compared to hierarchical bureaucracies and competitive markets.

At the conceptual level, Rhodes (2007) defines the term "network" as "sets of formal and informal institutional linkages between governmental and other actors structured around shared interests in public policymaking and implementation" (p. 1244). According to the above definition, network is a concept used to investigate non-centralized, horizontal, and interdependent relationships among various actors with a stake in policy making. The network approach has gained an increasingly significant position in public policy analysis for a minimum of two reasons. First, at the epistemological level, networks serve as tools to analyze the relational dimension of governance by investigating the practical or procedural side of policy making at the micro- and meso-level of analysis. Arguably, networks are particularly appropriate at the meso-level of analysis (Rhodes, 1990), which focuses on inter-organizational dynamics such as the relations between the government and interest groups, business organizations, or civil society organizations. At the ontological level, networks provide avenues to examine the collaborative side of policy by highlighting notions such as "joint governance," "shared experience," "joint problem solving," "joint action," "trust," and "reciprocity" (Laws & Hajer, 2006, p. 414). Within this framework, the network approach provides an opportunity to "deepen the account of cooperation" in public policy analysis compared to the other approaches in the literature that focus on "negotiation, conflict resolution and consensus building" (Laws & Hajer, 2006, p. 414).

Kenis and Schneider (1989) argue that policy networks were originally conceived as an inevitable response to contemporary political reality witnessed in advanced industrialized countries. Despite the extensive research done on the issue, following studies adhered to this axiom without heeding the mechanisms or conditions that lead to the preliminary emergence of networks. Isett and Provan (2005) assert that many scholars in the literature acknowledge the idea that networks emerge in turbulent policy environments in order to "manage uncertainty" and "smooth out operational flows" (p. 150). There is a general perception that networks are formed in policy areas characterized by dispersed costs and benefits, complexity in terms of the challenges being faced, innovation in terms of policy design, and uncertainty in terms of the outcomes. However, the specific ways through which networks emerge and influence policy processes have not been systematically evaluated through empirical research. As a result, starting from the second half of the 1990s, several key aspects of policy networks have been called into question and have come under increasing scrutiny.

One challenge addressed by Howlett (2002) has been to understand whether networks matter "in the sense of being a significant variable helping to understand, explain and predict policy outcomes" (p. 236). Moreover, since the 2000s, increasingly more scholars have called for case studies with findings translatable across research contexts, through the examination of the causal pathways that make network collaboration possible. Subsequently, there has been a soaring interest on the contextual conditions under which policy networks flourish and thrive in different policy settings across countries and even across policy sectors at the sub-national level. According to one account recorded by Kjaer (2011), a fully-fledged contextual analysis of networks should take into account the "social, economic and political parameters, including the nature of central and local state bureaucracy, strength of civil society, the organization of interests, and the traditions of state-society interaction" of the case under investigation (p. 111).

Following the rising criticisms in the field, the most recent research trends have been toward examining the contextual conditions favorable to the emergence, durability, and effectiveness of networks within policy processes that take place at the supra-national, national, and sub-national levels of governance. As a result, discussions in network research have developed in the direction of contextualization which implies generating systematic and thick descriptions about policy networks that can be extracted from countries other than the mature cases of network governance. In an attempt to contextualize networks, scholars have moved away from macro-level analysis toward more meso- and micro-level networks analysis. An increasing number of studies suggest that policy networks should no longer be treated as analytical tools to explain state-society or state-business relations at the macro-level of analysis. This approach leads to terminological confusion rather than clarity and provides no policy implications for practitioners. Instead, networks should be treated as policy tools relevant to policy processes and outcomes. According to Börzel (1998), network relevance to the practice of policy making can be constructed by empirically demonstrating the conditions that maximize network impact on policy processes and/or outcomes (e.g., effectiveness-driven policy). As described by DeLeon and Varda (2009), network relevance to policy may also be constructed by investigating the mechanisms that allow different stakeholders from the public, private, and voluntary sectors to participate in policy making processes (i.e., participation-driven approach). Despite the difference, these two approaches both suggest taking networks to the policy level of analysis.

This being the case, the main methodological challenge becomes adding explanatory power to the main methodological challenge explanatory power to the network concept so that it can be used to study those real world practices of policy making through empirical research. This entails constructing a network measure that would contribute to the operational dynamics of the concept. In their attempts to empirically investigate networks, Lewis (2011) asserts that researchers should combine "the structural and the processual aspects of networks [in order to] provide research space for interpretation without giving away causality" (p. 1232) through a synthesis of formal methods and interpretive methods. This logic brings us to middle-range theory which is particularly attentive to bridging empirical findings extracted from case studies, particularly with theoretical debates though a combination of inductive exploration and deductive explanation of the topic under investigation. According to Howlett (1991), middle-range theory is the most appropriate and reasonable approach in policy studies "subject to national variation and to broader conceptions and theorizations of national and international political life" (p. 13). Moreover, middle-range theory provides a set of practical tools to study forms of administrative responsiveness which, among others, include collaboration.

When applied to networks analysis, middle-range theory employs micro- and meso-level analysis of networks through the exploration of inter-personal and inter-organizational relationships, with the purpose of exploring the conditions favorable to the network mode of policy making. The findings generated through micro- and meso-level analysis can then be situated within a broader macro-level analysis that helps us explain the existing network categories within a given policy environment. This methodological choice sits well within Rhodes' approach according to which, "[p]olicy network is a meso-level concept which needs to be, and can be, located within very different macro-theoretical approaches" (1990, p. 309). Macro-level analysis seeks to identify dominant network policy making patterns at the system level which is neither possible nor useful considering that this approach prevents scholars from drawing variations within one country case (Rhodes, 1990). According to micro-analysis, on the other hand:

> Networks ... are constituted on the basis of informal relationships regulated by obligations of trust and reciprocity. Networks are frequently grounded in individual relationships that transcend organisational boundaries and even organisational agendas. They ... are fluid relationships that may grow up in response to a particular policy or service issue and will continue to operate for as long as the need exists and the network members are willing to sustain the relationship. (Sullivan & Skelcher, 2017, p. 5)

Micro-level analysis provides detailed accounts of policy networks as fluid actor configurations. The problem with this approach is that it "gives considerable weight to the role of individuals and individual personality; and raises the (perennial) problem of generalizability" (Rhodes, 1990, p. 310). Overall, integrating micro-, meso-, and macro-levels of analysis is useful to observe and compare network variations and offer middle-level generalizations. Considering the above discussion, this study seeks to formulate a middle-range conceptual framework for theorizing policy networks beyond Western liberal democracies.

Introducing Turkey to Network Research

Despite efforts to contextualize networks, not much is known about the practice of network policy making outside the context of advanced democracies, especially in low- and middle-income countries with perceived authoritarian predispositions. Scholars have highlighted the lack of and the need for the systematic and cross-national study of policy networks, including policy settings outside the context of advanced democracies (Kjaer, 2011; Klijn & Koppenjan, 2000; Klijn & Skelcher, 2007; O'Toole, 1997; Robichau, 2011). Limited empirical evidence and an absence of variation in terms of case selection have unquestionably hampered scholars from yielding broader generalizations concerning policy networks. Networks have often been criticized for remaining mere metaphors and theoretical notions rather than empirical tools (Börzel, 1998, 2011; Dowding, 1995, 2001; Dupont, 2006; Knox et al., 2006). More recent studies have reemphasized the lack of clarity in terms of network conceptualization and operationalization (Dal Molin & Masella, 2016; Lecy, Mergel, & Schmitz, 2014). In response to such criticisms, it becomes imperative to incorporate cross-national comparisons into the new research agenda on policy networks with a particular emphasis on empirical research in the context of low- and middle-income countries with governments that are increasingly likely to endorse an authoritarian attitude in policy making. Such comparisons are essential for laying out the theoretical foundations of networks as policy making instruments applicable across country cases.

Against this background, this book introduces Turkey as a middle-income country that has not been explored hitherto through the network perspective. Turkey has aspired to join the club of developed economies by emulating their policy models since 1980s, a goal that was more strongly restated after 2003 with the Justice and Development Party's (Adalet ve Kalkınma Partisi, AKP) rise to power. From a policy perspective, middle-income countries such as Turkey represent fertile ground for research considering that they have fast developing economies, dynamic societies, and governments that introduce major reform projects. Within the last 15 years, Turkey has undergone major structural transformations, particularly within the domain of health including the Health Transformation Programme (HTP) introduced in 2003.

Since the introduction of the HTP reforms, the Turkish health sector has made considerable progress. According to Sustainable Governance Indicators (SGI), health policy in Turkey displays a relatively high score compared to other social policies including education, social inclusion, family policy or pension policy (Genckaya,Togan, Schulz & Karadag, 2018). Relatively high levels of policy performance in the area of health have contributed to an improved health status among Turkish citizens. Recent OECD data show that Turkey has a relatively high score in terms of citizen health status, leaving behind other areas such as income and wealth, social connections, education and skills, jobs and earnings, subjective well-being, environmental quality, work-life balance, housing and personal security (OECD, 2017). Based on the above data, Turkey qualifies as a relatively high performer in the area of health.

From a governance perspective, the policy initiatives within the HTP reform package involve (a) multiple actors with a stake in policy making (e.g., multiplicity of actors in health tourism development); (b) various complex issues that require high levels of expertise and information sharing in terms of policy design (e.g., challenges in the context of public health policy development); and (c) and high levels of risk both in terms of the cost of policy implementation as well as the impact of the policy outcomes (e.g., risks involved in huge health construction projects). In the period from 2003 onwards, cross-sectoral arrangements that involve actors from the public, private, and voluntary sectors with a stake in health policy have increased significantly. Presently few descriptive studies have turned their attention toward cross-sectoral arrangements with the purpose of health policy making in Turkey (Dündar, 2018; Özkan, 2018; Pala, 2018). Even though these studies are informative of the current state of cross-sectoral collaboration taking place within the health sector, they do not examine the practical effectiveness and theoretical significance of these cases as novel policy instruments from a broader governance perspective.

The hesitation to study cross-sectoral collaboration from a broader governance perspective can partially be explained by emphasis put on authoritarian politics in Turkey. Recent political developments have sparked a scholarly interest toward *conflictual politics* with an emphasis on phenomena such as polarization of politics, populism, nationalism, and authoritarianism. Actually, in the last 10 years, there has been a growing debate on authoritarian or semi-authoritarian inclinations in Turkish politics. Hence, numerous studies have focused on the intersection between politics and authoritarianism mostly through the prism of political economy or state-society relations producing various hybrid categories such as competitive authoritarianism (Esen & Gümüşçü, 2016, 2018a; Özbudun, 2015), electoral authoritarianism (White & Herzog, 2016), hegemonic electoral authoritarianism (Esen & Gümüşçü, 2018b), new authoritarianism (Somer, 2016), authoritarian neoliberalism (Tansel, 2018), neoliberal populism (Akça, Bekmen, & Özden, 2014; Demiralp, 2018), illiberal governance (Öktem & Akkoyunlu, 2016), state capitalism, or authoritarian neo-developmentalism (Öniş, 2019). These accounts, to varying degrees and forms signal that the political regime is relapsing toward some sort of authoritarianism. Even though these studies paint a gloomy picture of Turkish politics, they should not preclude researchers from investigating the policy processes, particularly in those policy areas that involve new instruments and platforms of policy making.

The assumption here is that the presence of (semi)authoritarianism, even though is often presented as a linear regression back to more undemocratic and illiberal regime types, does not exclude participatory practices of policy making. This is especially the case in those formal yet unconsolidated democracies where governments come to power through elections, yet, demonstrate authoritarian predispositions mostly due to “the rapid rise of authoritarian-minded populist leaders” (Esen & Yardımcı-Geyikçi, 2019, p. 445). These countries, which do not fall in the diametrically opposed categories of western liberal democracies and the autarkic state, comprise of highly complex institutional and policy environments that remain largely undertheorized. Hence, new research should focus on explicating the dynamics of policy making within the broader political system in countries such as Turkey, particularly in the context of cross-cutting issues that require some degree of joint action manifested through various forms of cross-sectoral collaboration such as policy networks. Actually, Mahoney and Goertz (2004) would qualify Turkey as a negative case study, which can, and should be selected for comparative network research due to the possibility of network formation amid various cross-sectoral arrangements taking place within the health sector.

Despite its prominence, only a few studies have examined the new policy making patterns in Turkish politics (Atiyas & Bakış, 2015; Bölükbaşı & Ertuğal, 2018; Bölükbaşı, Ertuğal, & Özçürümez, 2018), but, even these studies are based upon macro-level institutional analysis which prioritizes the political and economic structures that shape policy making. One of the most ground-breaking studies in the field of public policy is the article published by Yıldız (2007) on e-government policy processes and actors. This study offers promising ground for advancing policy studies by linking “e-government research with those of newer research areas such as non-profit organizations, (policy) networks, third party government, governance, and globalization” (Yıldız, 2007, p. 661).

Considering limited research within the area of Turkish policy studies, this book suggests that more attention should be paid to the processes and procedures of policy making, which have been sidestepped due to almost exclusive attention put on political developments and administrative culture in Turkey. The case of Turkey presents new opportunities for the applicability of network concept through exploratory research at the micro- and meso-level of policy analysis. Being an essentially extreme case, a proper study of the Turkish case "refers back to a larger sample of cases lying in the background of the analysis" (Seawright & Gerring, 2008, p. 301) in an attempt to strike a balance between empirical findings from the ground and governance debates in the literature.

Following this logic, the main purpose of this book is to empirically examine the conditions under which existing policy networks emerge and thrive in Turkey, based on findings from the health policy sector. This examination is expected to develop a research agenda on cross-sectoral collaboration by assessing the context, capacity, and consequences of policy networks within the Turkish health sector covering the years between 2011 and 2015. To this end, this study is designed to provide sub-sectoral level comparison based on the investigation of network configurations within three health policy sub-areas: (a) public health, (b) health tourism, and (c) the medical industry. In addition, this study offers an account of the instances of cross-sectoral arrangements that fail to become collaborative. The essence of comparison across various cross-sectoral platforms is to assist researchers constructing variation at the sectoral and sub-sectoral levels of analysis. Finally, this book locates the cases under consideration within larger debates of governance guided by middle-range theory, which contributes to a better understanding of the concept and practice of the network type of collaboration.

The present study contributes to the academic debates on the variations and similarities in network policy making across country cases with implications for low- and middle-income countries where governments are increasingly likely to endorse an authoritarian attitude. This study contributes to network research through a micro- and meso-level investigation of policy networks. Following this approach, this book is expected to enrich and refine the debates on cross-sectoral collaboration drawing from the comparison of network configurations in three health policy sub-areas. As indicated in previous research "the comparison of policy areas at the sub-sectoral level is one of the more promising lines of research" in network analysis (Rhodes, 1990, p. 309). Through this exercise, this study represents an attempt to incorporate Turkey into the general debates of governance and serves the purpose of theory building based on a comparative case study investigation. "[E]mpirical and comparative case-study research" is considered to be a framework that should be followed by scholars of Turkish politics (Bölükbaşı, Ertuğal, & Özçürümez, 2010, p. 465). Case studies are becoming increasingly important by providing "thick, rich descriptive accounts" which can be used to "triangulate the results of large-N studies that we are increasingly using in network research" (Berry et al., 2004, p. 549).

In addition, the book represents an attempt to incorporate network analysis into the debates on health governance in the context of developing countries. The area of health policy provides fertile ground for the emergence of networks and as a result has become one of the main domains of research in network analysis, particularly in advanced democracies (Greenaway, Salter, & Hart, 2007; Huang & Provan, 2006, 2007; Isett & Provan, 2005; Kenis & Provan, 2009; Lewis, 2006; Meyer & Scheepers, 2017; Provan, Huang, & Milward, 2009; Provan, Isett, & Milward, 2004; Provan & Kenis, 2008; Provan & Milward, 1995, 1999; Provan, Milward, & Isett, 2002; Raab & Milward, 2003; Tenbensel, Cumming, Ashton, & Barnett, 2008; Tenbensel, Mays, & Cumming, 2011). Recently, health governance has become an increasingly important issue in the agenda of developmental politics as well, particularly due to the pressures placed by international actors such as the World Health Organization (WHO). WHO has supported different forms of collaborative governance in low- and middle-income countries particularly in but not confined to the areas primary health services and community-based healthcare services (Best et al., 2018, Dickerson, Grills, Henwood, Jeffreys, & Lankester, 2012; Pyone, Smith, & van den Broek, 2017). This book offers concrete policy implications for developing countries that are actively pursuing health system reforms by focusing on those horizontal and networked forms of governance that stipulate interaction among stakeholders within the health sector. Within this framework, this book aims at building a link between health governance and developmental politics, through the study of network policy making in Turkey.

Ultimately, this book contributes to the studies on Turkish politics, particularly public policy and public administration debates. The majority of the studies in Turkish politics deal extensively with the issues of political and economic structure or administrative culture sidestepping even important policy issues. Yıldız and Babaoğlu (2018) note that until very recently, systematic studies on public policy in Turkey were virtually missing, leading to the "inability of public policy studies to become an autonomous academic discipline in Turkey" (p. 282). According to this study policy related research articles were observed after the second half of 2000s, especially since 2010s. However, in the last 10 years public policy research in Turkey pays almost exclusive attention to statist policy making patterns through the study of purported *heroic policies*, such as macro-economy, foreign policy, and national security – thus overshadowing *everyday policies* such as social inclusion, health, and education (see Bölükbaşı & Ertuğal, 2018, for the usage of the terms heroic and everyday policies). Against this background, this examination aims at filling this gap in the literature by investigating policy networks as a new area of research in public administration and public policy in Turkish studies.

Finally, this study represents an attempt to examine the role of societal actors in policy processes in Turkish politics, through a detailed assessment of expert (professional associations, business associations, and specialized NGOs) involvement in policy making. As maintained by Heper (1993), both societal elites and state elites are expected to play an active role toward policy making "in the name of 'general interest'" in a way "that reflects the notion of liberal-democratic state" (pp. 16–17). Studies of the Turkish case have shown that societal actors have traditionally had minimal or no impact on public policy making due to impediments such as populism, clientelism, and opportunism (Heper & Yıldırım, 2011). In this context, networks can be perceived as important channels of societal participation, more specifically expert involvement in policy making processes, as well as, tools that deliver policy legitimacy which is at the heart of public policy issues. In this way, through the study of networks within the health sector in Turkey, this book contributes to the debates on widening participation in policy making processes, with implications for policy legitimacy in the developing countries.

Doing Field Research in an Unexplored Territory: Data, Methods, and Analysis

The researcher was confronted with many challenges during the preparation of this book, which aims at framing research questions and designing a research protocol in an unexplored territory. The most challenging task has been to provide a clear definition that guides the investigation of networks on the ground in a focused and systematic fashion which excludes any ambiguous cases of cross-sectoral arrangements discussed in the literature. In this study, networks are defined as cross-sectoral platforms (interaction among public, private, and voluntary actors) that facilitate collaboration in a repetitive fashion over a relatively extended time period (purposeful, repeated, and systematic as opposed to ad hoc, sporadic, or spontaneous interaction) with the purpose of policy making (interaction that shapes public policy to varying degrees and forms). This definition implies that policy networks do not simply influence policies through indirect channels such as engaging in activism, attending ad hoc meetings or policy workshops, lobbying through interest groups, or exerting leverage via political parties in the legislature. Instead, the definition demonstrates that policy networks shape policies through cross-sectoral platforms that facilitate some degree of collaborative interaction public, private, and voluntary actors at different stages of policy making from policy formulation to policy evaluation. Theoretically, this definition situates networks within broader theories of collaborative policy making. Practically, it helps the researcher distinguish policy networks from other cross-sectoral interactions that fail to become collaborative.

This network definition has been utilized to examine various practices of cross-sectoral interaction across three policy sub-areas within the health sector in the post-2003 period in Turkey. The data collected during field research consist of (a) semi-structured interviews with professional experts and policy makers in the respective policy sub-areas (March–December 2015); (b) field notes, informal talks with healthcare practitioners and policy makers, and audio-recorded speeches delivered in the 3rd Convention on Healthcare Management (Ankara, April 13–16, 2015)[1]; and (c) field notes and audio-recorded speeches from the monthly meeting organized by the Turkish Medicines and Medical Devices Agency (TMMDA, July 1, 2015).[2] The majority of the information presented

[1]3. Sağlık Yönetimi Kongresi Nisan 2015/Ankara https://www.medikalakademi.com.tr/kongre/3-saglik-yonetimi-kongresi/

[2]The Medical Devices Meeting was arranged within the building of the *Turkish Medicines and Medical Devices Agency* on July 1, 2015. The meeting took place behind closed doors with attendance by invitation only.

in the following chapters was derived from content analysis of the interview transcripts. Other encounters in the field were useful to learn about key health policy issues concerning critical policy decisions, current legislative framework, in addition to important actor constellations, including key figures in the central and local government, and prominent stakeholder groups in the respective policy areas. These encounters in the field helped the researcher determine the main issues of concern and enhance access to the main affiliation networks within the health sector. Attending these conferences introduced the researcher to those policy sub-areas with enriched cross-sectoral interaction and correspondingly contributed toward building the sample of network involved actors.

The first step of field research was sample selection. An accurate network analysis requires a careful sample design which will target the right constellation of actors. Purposive, non-random sampling techniques suit this type of research best. In this case, the researcher is not interested in the whole population but only in those professional experts who represent organizations that have been actively involved in cross-sectoral arrangements and/or who are competent enough to give rich information on those arrangements. Interviews have been conducted with professional experts from the public, private, and voluntary sectors, who have been or are still involved in cross-sectoral projects in the fields of (a) public health development, (b) health tourism, and (c) medical industry. In more concrete terms, experts interviewed here are either high-level officials or mid-level government experts who have knowledge in policy making as well as internal and external stakeholder relations or professionals working in the private and voluntary sectors who have some accumulated knowledge in their respective fields as well as experience in cross-sectoral projects.

Expert interviews utilized in this study are as Littig (2009) suggests a specific form of elite interviewing "aimed at generating explicit, tacit, professional or occupational knowledge" (p. 99). The main rationale behind using expert interviews reflects the purpose of the study itself. As stated in the previous research of Onwuegbuzie and Leech (2007):

> [i]f the goal is not to generalize to a population but to obtain insights into a phenomenon, individuals, or events … then the researcher purposefully selects individuals, groups, and settings that maximize understanding of the phenomenon. (p. 111)

Doing expert interviews for policy network research is justified for two practical reasons. First and foremost, the nature of the items included in the questionnaire is more suitable for professional experts who have specialized knowledge in the field. Secondly, expert interviews are often used in qualitative and explorative studies in order to provide orientations in new fields of research (Bogner, Littig, & Menz, 2009).

Professional experts were selected through a multistage purposeful sampling (see Collins, Onwuegbuzie, & Jiao, 2006 for sampling designs) where the selection of interviewees follows a careful procedure of two or more stages rather than a one-time decision. Here, sampling involves selection of actors in two stages.

The objective of the first stage is to select those actors who are willing to contribute to health policy making (e.g., sample of politically relevant actors) amidst numerous actors operating within the health sector. Politically relevant actors refer to those private/voluntary organizations and public/semi-public agencies that identify themselves declared as politically active and literally state on their official websites that they are interested in and willing to contribute to the development of health policy making. Politically relevant actors were identified through desk research. The objective of the second stage is to filter actors from the first sample based on their actual involvement into cross-sectoral arrangements within the three specified policy areas (e.g., sample of network involved actors). Field research guided the development of the sample of network involved actors, through the techniques of pilot interviewing and modified snowballing.

The first pilot interviews were held with bureaucrats from the Health Investments Directorate, at the Ministry of Health in March 2015. Pilot interviews conducted with policy experts from the Ministry of Health are of crucial importance to collect information on respondents' views and opinions, to review and refine the interview questions, and to receive some information about which organizations should be included or excluded from the sample of actors to be investigated through modified snowballing. Based on such information, a series of semi-structured interviews with experts working in the public sector was carried out in the following eight months. During the interview process, respondents were asked about significant other actors to make sure the right connections were identified and the right network participants were interviewed. One of the biggest challenges of this study was to estimate a sufficient sample size which would fulfill both criteria of data saturation and in-depth information.

This study is essentially exploratory research for policy analysis which means that the sample should be large enough to give us adequate information, but at the same time, small enough to provide rich, in depth information (Onwuegbuzie & Leech, 2007, p. 116). Existing methodological studies recommend interviewing between 15–20 people, 20–30 people, and 30–50 people in grounded theory research (Creswell, 1998; Morse, 1994, 2000). The target in this study was to reach out to an average of 20–30 experts which can be considered sufficient in terms of inter-expert agreement and data saturation. Another criterion was to keep an equal number of participants between state actors (e.g., public and semi-public actors) on the one hand and non-state actors (e.g., private and voluntary actors) on the other hand. In total, 24 interviews were audio taped, transcribed, and included in the analysis. The sample includes 12 interviewees working in the ministerial or other government-related offices. Representing non-governmental organizations from the private and voluntary sectors are 12 other interviewees. Open-ended questions with sub-questions recorded by the researcher were utilized during the interview, corresponding to categories and sub-categories used in the analysis of the transcripts.

Content analysis was utilized to examine and categorize the information retrieved from interview transcripts. The advantage of content analysis is that it allows the researcher to combine both quantitative and qualitative techniques through different types of coding. It is worth mentioning here that qualitative analysis is triggering more and more interest in policy studies particularly when coupled with quantitative analysis. This is mostly due to the growing complexity of issues and phenomena being investigated. According to Ritchie and Spencer (2002), qualitative research is regaining prominence in the field of social sciences and particularly policy analysis in order to "explore and understand a diversity of social and public policy issues, either as an independent research strategy or in combination with some form of statistical inquiry" (p. 173). Bryman and Burgess (2002) argue that coding is the most critical aspect of content analysis as it represents not only the categorization or classification of data in a systematic fashion, but also the "link between data and conceptualization" (p. 5). The type of coding employed in this examination refers to "the coding of open-ended questions ... where the aim is to quantify different categories of a variable" (Bryman & Burgess, 2002, p. 5). Categories and corresponding sub-categories have been constructed and refined by the researcher in a gradual fashion during the field research process in order to measure network collaborative capacity index (NCC). The same set of categories are applied across the whole dataset based on the principle cross-sectional categorical indexing. According to Mason (2002), the purpose of cross-sectional categorical indexing is to analyze text-based data in a consistent, systematic, and comparable fashion (pp. 150–151). At the end of this process, qualitative data extracted from the interview texts are quantified (e.g., they are assigned numerical values corresponding to categories and sub-categories included in content analysis). Finally, the numerical values of all categories are aggregated at the network level in order to measure overall collaborative capacity of each policy network.

The technique of quantifying qualitative data was first introduced in 1997 as quantitative-based qualitative approach or verbal analysis which Chi (1997) maintains aims at "operationaliz[ing] one's subjective impression by coding the verbal evidence for that impression and comparing the frequencies of the codes quantitatively" (p. 282). Categories have been coded through literal and interpretative reading of the transcript data. Literal categories reflect descriptive, straightforward information without any need for interpretation on the side of the researcher. Interview questions used to measure these categories inquire relatively technical information such as "types of organizations involved in the cross-sectoral arrangements under investigation." Quantification of literal categories is a direct calculation of the numerical values assigned to corresponding sub-categories put on a 0–1 scale. Interpretative categories, alternatively, are built upon explanations, opinions, or judgments of the interviewees and can hardly be measured through fixed criteria and require some engagement on the part of the researcher. Similar to the literal categories described above, they can still be applied across data and they can be quantified; however, this process is relatively more sophisticated and requires the researcher to exercise caution. For instance, *trust* can take several forms at the inter-personal and inter-organizational level within a network. The trust category and sub-categories can be calculated through quantified measures based on an interpretative reading of the text. Considering the challenges of coding, some interpretative categories such as *inter-personal level trust* are measured as either 0 (present) or 1 (absent).

Scholars including Green (2001) have indicated skepticism about the extent to which qualitative data, often used in social science disciplines, can produce reliable quantitative findings. Combination of quantitative and qualitative methods seems to be a source of concern particularly for researchers investigating health-related topics, with repercussions for the society at large (Bryman, 2007). Taking into account these concerns, this study makes use of the technique of inter-expert agreement which was utilized during content analysis to quantify both the literal and interpretative categories. The researcher focuses on the responses where experts are in agreement with each other. For example, if several respondents referring to the same project reiterate words such "team work," "synergy," and "collaborative spirit," the researcher records an advanced level of trust at the inter-organizational level which is then quantified on a 0 to 1 scale based on the specified sub-categories. Previous research has found that "it makes intuitive sense to use agreement among experts as an indication of the quality of the information they provided" (Dorussen, Lenz, & Blavoukos, 2005, p. 318). The extent of agreement has been larger than disagreement on the issues of concern which adds reliability to the findings. Lastly, the transcript data were coded and recoded several times during the field research in order to add to the validity of the constructed categories and sub-categories used in the analysis.

Book Organization

This section briefly summarizes the content of the chapters included in this book. Chapter 2 outlines the mechanisms that encourage network collaboration among several stakeholders based on the existing debates within the policy networks/governance networks literature. The purpose of this chapter is to construct a comprehensive, yet parsimonious integrated framework that can be utilized to study networks across policy settings and country cases. This framework incorporates structural, relational, and institutional mechanisms which can be combined to produce different causal pathways of network collaboration depending on the case under investigation. The remainder of the book has an essentially explorative design tailored to shed light on various aspects of cross-sectoral collaboration through the empirical investigation and analytical evaluation of network policy making within the Turkish health sector. The following chapters contribute toward a common understanding of network policy making within the Turkish health sector, but they can also be read separately as accounts that target different aspects of network collaboration, namely, the origins of network formation (Chapter 3), mechanisms that enhance network collaboration (Chapter 4), factors that impede network collaboration (Chapter 5), and theoretical and practical significance of existing policy networks (Conclusion).

Chapter 3 investigates network formation by addressing the questions of *when* and *why* policy networks emerge. In an attempt to answer these questions, this chapter combines information derived from desk and field research. This chapter provides an overview of the cooperative policy processes within the Turkish health policy system focusing on the aftermath of 2003, a turning point that corresponds to the introduction of the HTP, and offers a narrative of the origins of policy networks within the health sector as innovative policy instruments that involve cross-sectoral collaboration with an impact on policy making processes and outcomes concentrated in the period between 2011 and 2015. As expected, the following questions asked in this study are the following: What are the critical junctures that led to the establishment of collaborative platforms with the purpose of policy making particularly after 2011 within the health sector in Turkey? In a similar vein, what caused the slow-down of cross-sectoral collaboration in the aftermath of 2015?

Chapter 4 further advances the debate on policy networks by examining the conditions that maximize collaboration based on the findings of the field research conducted in the period between March and December 2015 in Turkey. Here, structural capacity, relational capacity, and institutional capacity of three policy networks and their impact on networks' overall capacity to collaborate is investigated. Findings reveal that each policy network represents a distinct model of policy making with varying levels of collaborative capacity. Sub-sectoral level comparison offered in this chapter suggests the presence of variation in network collaboration at the national level. Furthermore, this chapter highlights the comparative advantages and disadvantages of each type of network collaboration by drawing a parallel with similar network practices witnessed in advanced democracies. Finally, this chapter suggests the importance of incorporating neo-institutionalist approaches to network analysis, particularly in the context of low- and middle-income countries with constantly shifting political, economic, and social circumstances.

Chapter 5 unpacks the structural and cultural impediments that hinder the development of network collaboration by focusing on those cross-sectoral arrangements that fail to become collaborative. Three instances of failed collaboration will be elaborated in this chapter, namely, consultative networks, cluster networks, and patronage networks. This account is necessary to distinguish policy networks from other cross-sectoral arrangements with no genuine network dynamics in addition to providing insights for similar country cases that face similar policy challenges. Chapter 4 suggests that policy collaboration is not an inherent quality of networks, which can reverse to structures that hide clientelist and asymmetrical power relations or give way to further fragmentation among loosely connected stakeholders.

Finally, the concluding chapter offers a brief discussion of the theoretical and practical significance of network policy making based on the findings from the Turkish health sector. The goal here is to assess the impact that networks have on policy making processes and/or outcomes as well as the political system at large. The cases elaborated in this study show that networks have the potential to enhance policy innovation especially at the phase of policy formulation; organizational-knowledge-sharing at the inter-phase between policy formulation and policy implementation; and policy effectiveness through co-production at the phase of policy implementation. This examination suggests rising to the challenge of cross-sectoral collaboration by leveraging networks as instruments of collaborative policy making. Lastly, this chapter discusses some limitations of the present study and offers suggestions for future research on the issue of policy networks, particularly through the elaboration of the term network resilience in dynamic, yet, often unpredictable policy environments.

Chapter 2

Setting the Stage: An Integrated Framework for Assessing Network Collaboration Across Country Cases

Abstract

This chapter provides a comprehensive, yet, concise overview of the existing debates on policy networks. The aim of the chapter is to identify those mechanisms that encourage network collaboration among several stakeholders with different motivations, interests, and preferences throughout different stages of policy making from agenda setting to policy evaluation. A systematic review of previous studies on policy networks across various countries highlights the achievements and missing links in the literature, and at the same time, reveals three sets of causal mechanisms, which are crucial to understand Network Collaborative Capacity (NCC) along the structural, relational, and institutional dimensions. Structural and relational mechanisms explain the internal dynamics of a policy network; whereas institutional mechanisms consist of all those external factors in the broader political and economic environment within which the network is embedded. Structural, relational, and institutional mechanisms are further classified into constituting elements that serve as a blueprint for organizing and managing collaborative efforts at the network level. Ultimately this chapter contributes to the existing governance debates by offering an integrated framework for the study of NCC across country cases and policy sectors. Turkish health sector represents a case study to assess the applicability of this framework beyond the context of advanced industrialized economies and democracies with a tradition in collaborative policy making. Finally, the added value of comparative network analysis at the national and subnational levels will be discussed.

Keywords: Collaborative capacity; institutionalization; integrated framework; network structure; policy networks; trust

Network Policy Making within the Turkish Health Sector: Becoming Collaborative, 17–40

doi:10.1108/978-1-83867-094-820201003

> Since the time of Aristotle, the first task of comparison is to observe the extent to which countries differ or are similar. The second task is to ask why. Under what circumstances do differences occur? Particularly in policy studies, a third question is also significant: what are the consequences of observed differences? (Rose & Mackenzie, 1991, p. 447)

Policy networks are placed in a bizarre situation. On the one hand, they are studied as a phenomenon peculiar to countries with an established tradition of policy collaboration – almost unique to advanced democracies. On the other hand, they are assumed to be inevitable developments of the contemporary political regimes – almost ubiquitous phenomena present across country cases and policy areas. However, as Richard Rose and William J. M. Mackenzie (1991) bring to our attention, "[t]he study of comparative politics rejects the extremes of universalism and particularism; it assumes what may be termed 'bounded variability'" (p. 447). When translated to network analysis, this statement compels researchers to investigate conditions under which policy networks emerge and thrive based on established and widely recognized criteria of comparison across country cases as well as policy sectors.

The aim of this chapter is to unravel mechanisms that facilitate collaboration at the network level in an attempt to go beyond the present body of work that builds almost exclusively upon mature cases of network governance. Here, mechanisms refer to those processes and procedures that encourage collaborative capacity at the network level, that is, Network Collaborative Capacity (NCC). It is important to emphasize that mechanisms of network collaboration are not be treated as variables in a conventional sense. This epistemological shift from variables to mechanisms corresponds to the recently discussed shift from meta-theories (of universal application) to contextually situated approaches (Falleti & Lynch, 2009). In the former case, the factors (independent variables) associated with policy collaboration at the network level (dependent variable) would be examined. The goal of this analysis would be to build direct causal links that predict higher levels of network collaboration regardless of the country and policy context. In the latter case, mechanisms gain validity depending on the contextual conditions under investigation; a situation Rose and Mackenzie (1991) would call bounded variability. While some of the conditions are critical in organizing collaborative efforts within networks, some of them might be completely absent. In this case, the question becomes: Under what conditions is network collaboration maximized in different policy settings? Following this logic, different causal pathways (combination of different causal mechanisms) can lead to different types and degrees of network collaboration depending largely upon the policy setting under investigation.

The rest of the chapter is structured as follows: The first section is an overview of the two main ontological and epistemological approaches to policy networks. The second section is a critique of the literature focusing on some of the gaps in the study of policy networks. The third section introduces an integrated framework for the study of policy networks across country cases and policy settings, based on a synthesis of the previous debates on policy networks and in an attempt to fill in the gaps in the literature. The final section provides some concluding remarks on the applicability of the suggested framework to different policy settings at the national and sub-national level.

Policy Networks: Two Dominant Approaches

An extensive review of some of the studies on network-type policy collaboration shows that two approaches have dominated the literature, namely: the network governance approach (governance perspective to networks), and the institutionalist approach (policy perspective to networks), which constitute two different ontological positions on policy networks.

As the name indicates, the network governance approach, associated with the Network Governance School (NGS), refers to policy networks as a discrete form of collaborative governance next to competitive markets and hierarchical bureaucracies. This approach focuses more on the internal dynamics of policy networks, with particular attention to the nature of intra-network interaction. The network governance approach consists of a normative approach and a functionalist approach to networks. To start with, the normative approach considers policy networks as the prominent governance paradigm. According to this approach, the conceptual distinction between policy networks and governance networks (and eventually network governance) can be rejected. Both these networks feed each other and are in a way both following the same logic of governing, same motive, same ethos, that is, joint problem solving. Instead of "policy networks" one can as well use the terms "networked services" or "network system" (Rethemeyer & Hatmaker, 2007). Policy networks are not simply a policy instrument; they constitute a pattern of governance which serves as a bridge between state and society through increased involvement of private and voluntary actors in policy making. This makes policy networks a highly valuable and desirable form of governing compared to other more traditional forms such as hierarchies or markets.

The notion of network governance has attracted a lot of attention among scholars of various disciplines due to its primary concern with the involvement of private and voluntary actors in policy making. It is due to this feature that policy networks represent a substantial break from the traditional governing mechanisms and a new pattern of governance (Rhodes, 1996, 1997, 2007; Sørensen, 2002, 2005, 2006; Sørensen & Torfing, 2005, 2007, 2009, 2016; Stoker, 1998, 2006). The debate on network governance has been spurred by the work of Rod Rhodes based on the changes that took place in British politics starting from the second half of the 1980s. Gerry Stoker (1998) develops this argument further by claiming that policy networks "involve not just influencing government policy but taking over the business of government" (p. 23). Eva Sørensen and Jacob Torfing (2007) introduce a more elaborate definition of policy networks as "relatively institutionalized frameworks of negotiated interaction within which different actors struggle with each other, create opportunities for joint decisions, forge political compromises and coordinate concrete actions" (p. 27).

The original definition of policy networks, that is, to some degree, still used today describes networks as "self-organizing, inter-organizational networks characterized by 1) interdependence, 2) resource-exchange, 3) rules of the game, and 4) significant autonomy from the state" (Rhodes, 1997, p. 15). First of all, network members involved in governance are dependent upon each other for resources. Secondly, network members involved in governance are in continuous interaction with each other in order to exchange resources and to achieve their shared policy goals. Thirdly, network members involved in governance employ strategies within the known rules of the game negotiated and decided by network participants. Finally, policy networks enjoy a significant degree of autonomy from the state (not accountable to the state), which gives these networks a self-governing nature. What makes this approach essentially normative is the assumption that policy networks consist of multiple public, private, and voluntary actors, which are distinct from other traditional forms of governance, and they are better equipped to cope with new policy challenges. Such networks "complement markets and hierarchies as governing structures for authoritatively allocating resources and exercising control and co-ordination" (Rhodes, 1996, p. 652). Unlike markets and hierarchies, which are characterized by competition and authority, respectively, networks are characterized by relations of trust, interdependence, and reciprocity (Rhodes, 1996), which make policy networks inherently better instruments of policy making.

Not all scholars agree on this point. According to the functionalist or rationalist approach, the inclusive, interdependent, and reciprocal nature of network interaction does not automatically turn it into a superior form of governance. At the end of the day, policy networks are instruments of policy making and should be treated as such. The assumption here is a functionalist one, that is, networks are useful instruments of governance because they contribute to effective policy making – namely, problem amelioration through improved coordination among actors, greater coherence, and synergy. Networks are useful instruments of policy making rather than the best model of governance to be pursued invariably.

Scholars from the German school of thought follow the functionalist/rationalist approach to policy networks. In one of his research articles Jörg Raab (2002) hypothesizes that the "comparative advantages of networks in specific situations" (p. 582) is one factor that contributes to the development of policy networks. His findings suggest that networks offer better coping strategies under certain challenging circumstances. Such coping strategies involve "intense (informal) communication with a high information load, mobilization of diverse knowledge, and trust relationships" among various actors (Raab, 2002, p. 619). Following this logic, networks emerge as solutions in specific policy settings. Therefore, the study of policy networks entails a detailed study of policy making processes, actors, and outcomes. Study of policy processes is usually carried out at the sectoral or subsectoral level in order to measure the concrete policy impact of networks on policy making – replacing those studies that focus on state-society relations in general.

Both normative and functionalist approaches highlight the comparative advantages of policy networks over other forms of governing, which has been very useful in the study of policy networks in the so-called network pioneer countries. However, the network features that these authors discuss are not necessarily transferrable and applicable beyond the boundaries of those "ideal" cases of network governance, which is the weakest point in these debates.

The NGS has been criticized by the institutionalist camp, which highlights the loose institutionalist dimension of networks as fluid structures. According to institutionalist approaches, policy networks do not really constitute a paradigm shift or a *sui generis* form of governing in the context of governance debates. This approach acknowledges that policy networks, as concepts and practices, are worth the attention of scholars. However, they do not necessarily represent a new stage of governance. Scholars following institutionalist approaches advocate the argument that new forms of governance, including network governance, are not really "new" (as they existed before in the form of policy networks), and they have not replaced the traditional forms of governing (Blanco, Lowndes, & Pratchett, 2011; Jordan, Wurzel, & Zito, 2005; Knill & Lehmkuhl, 2002; Olsen, 2005; Parker, 2007; Richardson, 2000).

The concerns of institutionalists derive from their epistemological position, which pays particular attention to the emergence and maintenance of structures. The presence of various forms of policy networks does not necessarily indicate the emergence of new forms of governance (Blanco, Lowndes, & Pratchett, 2011; Parker, 2007). For network governance to represent a "turn" in policy studies, networks should have specific structural characteristics that influence the behavior of their participants and result in the pursuit of collective goals (Parker, 2007, p. 118). Otherwise, networks are simply neologisms for old forms of governing. For instance, Jeremy Richardson (2000) notes that the process of governance has always involved using networks of some kind, so we should not exclusively focus our attention on policy networks in our studies (p. 1021). He argues that the concepts such as policy network and community are useful in studying recent developments of governance and policy making. But the presence of policy networks or communities does not necessarily lead to the emergence of network governance. In addition, Richardson draws our attention to the malleability and flexibility of policy networks, which can, in a way, make them vulnerable structures. He argues that factors such as constantly changing ideas and knowledge often upset the structure of policy networks. To substantiate his argument, he gives the example of networks at the EU level (the EU is providing new fora for networks and policy communities to get involved in policy making) which he describes as uncertain agendas, shifting networks, and complex coalitions (due to factors outside the network dynamics themselves, i.e., external factors). He suggests that we pay particular attention to actors' changing ideas over time because such changes are also reflected in the rules and power distribution of the networks and policy communities (Richardson, 2000, p. 1022).

Another type of research refers to policy networks as institutional arrangements that bring together actors who hold different interests and policy strategies at the domestic level. These institutional arrangements reflect the power relations between the involved actors. In this case, power is the defining criterion that distinguishes different governing types, which can vary from strong governance to strong government (Jordan, Wurzel, & Zito, 2005). Governance and government are two ideal types, or "poles on a continuum of different governing types" (Jordan et.al., 2005, p. 480). The cases in between them are "hybrid types" which consist of a different network arrangement that serves as channels of interest intermediation between societal and governmental actors (see the typology suggested by Jordan et al., 2005). In the same vein, policy networks serve as concepts that are utilized to analyze state-business relations (Van Waarden, 1992).

According to institutionalist approaches discussed above, policy networks are fluid institutional arrangements where different actors, interests, and strategies meet. They can take different forms depending on the power distribution between governmental and non-governmental actors. In this way, institutional typologies are useful for analyzing and comparing different forms of power distribution within a polity, particularly in the context of state-business and state-civil society relations. However, networks have no one distinct and stable structure that distinguishes them as a discrete pattern of governance, which makes comparison across countries quite challenging. Besides, within the institutionalist framework, "policy networks" runs the risk of turning into a heuristic device used to analyze a wide range of institutional arrangements, power relations, and actors configurations, without constituting an entity of its own.

The Missing Element in Network Research

As mentioned above, the study of networks has become an indispensable part of the body of research on policy making. The network governance approaches have been useful in identifying elements pertaining to intra-network structure and relations. Institutional perspectives have been more concerned with the extra-network actor constellations, power relations, and sets of ideas that shape networks as policy undertakings. Whether they represent a new stage in governance or not, the study of policy networks contributes to the understanding of the organizational or procedural dimension of policy making by investigating how relevant actors connect to each other from the stage of policy inception to the stage of policy implementation. Yet, understanding the conditions under which policy networks emerge and thrive has not proved that easy. In a similar vein, the study of issues pertaining to network consequences, such as effectiveness, innovation, accountability, or the contribution of networks to some sort of democratic policy making remains challenging.

Besides the challenges mentioned above, the concept of network collaboration has only entered the political vocabulary of advanced industrialized economies such as Canada, the USA, the UK, continental Europe, New Zealand, and Australia. Most of the research so far takes the form of single case studies of countries mentioned above or theoretical debates with no empirical evidence. To date, relatively few studies have chosen to conduct comparative research at the cross-national level (Atkinson & Coleman, 1989; Coleman, Skogstad, & Atkinson, 1996; Considine & Lewis, 2003; Haveri, Nyholm, Roiseland, & Vabo, 2009; Kenis, Marin, & Mayntz, 1991). Similarly, few studies have examined policy networks outside the original context of advanced industrialized economies (Brass, 2012; Fulda, Li, & Song, 2012; Gebara, Fatorelli, May, & Zhang, 2014; Shiroma, 2014; Shrestha, 2012; Zheng, De Jong, & Koppenjan, 2010). It goes without saying that policy networks as conceptual tools have largely remained in the context they first emerged often referred to as network pioneer countries.

The sample of advanced industrialized countries with an already pluralistic policy environment is far from being representative, as it excludes those developing countries with traditionally centralized policy making within authoritarian regimes or "softer" variations that take the form of semi-authoritarianism, competitive authoritarianism, or electoral authoritarianism. These regime types, standing between authoritarianism and democracy, are not only on the rise but also represent models of dynamic institutional change, opening up new lines of research in network analysis. So far, the UK has been considered the ideal or the authoritative case for the study of policy networks among scholarly circles. Other countries are either "close" or "far" from this ideal case, with no clear and standard criteria of comparison across country cases. Despite extensive research done on the issue of policy networks, lack of clarity about the criteria of comparison has resulted in inadequate cross-country variation – adding to the conceptual confusion surrounding policy networks.

Limited empirical evidence, inadequate cross-country variation, and confusion over criteria of comparison across cases have certainly hampered scholars from yielding broader generalizations concerning policy networks. Present "research draws conclusions from empirical studies in particular temporal, spatial and political contexts" (Klijn & Skelcher, 2007, p. 605). The countries studied so far are characterized by consensual governmental norms and greater local autonomy. But conclusions drawn from these country studies should not be directly applied to countries with more antagonistic cultures and highly centralized policy making (Klijn & Skelcher, 2007). Even if the organizing principles of governance have a global scope, application of findings on policy networks to "multiple contexts can sharpen controversy" (Robichau, 2011, p. 116). Obviously, scholars recognize the lack of a comparative framework that would enable the study of policy networks outside the context of industrialized and advanced democracies.

First, the lack of a comparative framework can be attributed to the difficulty of concurring with a general and abstract category or, perhaps, an "umbrella concept" that explains the instances of network collaboration researchers investigate. The confusion at the theoretical level is partially due to the plethora of cases that researchers encounter in their empirical investigations. The studies show that there are diverse forms of "networking" experienced differently in different social, economic, and political contexts. Even when similar network configurations are observed, contextual conditions under which such networks emerge vary across policy settings. Scholars have been primarily preoccupied with studying upper income countries – a sample of states with similar contexts. By keeping the contextual factors constant, existing studies do not provide much theoretical insight or practical implications for policy settings outside the advanced democracies. This compels us to go a step further and explore the factors that produce such variety in the first place, by comparing different policy settings across country cases or within the same country but across policy areas.

Second, by taking the phenomenon of network collaboration for granted, the primary goal in the existing literature has been to trace the evolution of the existing policy networks rather than explore the causal mechanisms that foster collaboration within networks once they are formed. In the context of advanced democracies, researchers presume the presence of equal power relations among a web of politically and economically interdependent actors with a stake in policy making as well as the presence of organizational structures that facilitate a symmetrical or horizontal interaction among them. In addition, researchers presume the existence of high levels of social capital that motivates non-state actors to get involved in cross-sectoral policy making processes. Such deeply seated structural factors are often lumped together and their presence is taken for granted in the context of network governance pioneers. Hence, a comparative framework that would integrate various mechanisms applicable across policy settings is absent.

The argument here is that network research should account for both contextual conditions and causal mechanisms that foster network policy making, particularly in those countries which have not witnessed a substantial shift toward consensual, decentralized, and pluralistic forms of governance. This research design requires more empirically grounded and comparative studies, particularly in those under-researched contexts characterized by antagonistic cultures and traditionally centralized policy making environments. Turkey falls within this category of countries and consequently constitutes a crucial case study. Crucial cases "can be quite powerful tools to test and/unpack an existing theory and come up with new, better arguments about causal mechanisms" (Hancké, 2009, p. 61) and consequently contribute to theory building. The purpose of this chapter is to examine policy networks within the Turkish health sector through an integrated framework, which incorporates contextual conditions and causal mechanisms that foster network collaboration at the policy level. While contextual conditions are specific to the case under consideration, the rest of this chapter provides a discussion of the causal mechanisms that can maximize NCC across country cases.

Introducing an Integrated Framework for Assessing Network Collaboration

According to the definition outlined in Chapter 1 of the book, networks refer to platforms that involve cross-sectoral collaboration among public, private, and voluntary actors with some measurable impact on policy making processes and/or outcomes. By definition, policy networks have three constituting elements: (a) network interaction takes place within regularly arranged platforms rather than sporadic occurrences or intermittent meetings among stakeholders; (b) network interaction is regulated by the principle of collaboration, more specifically cross-sectoral collaboration among public, private, and voluntary actors, rather than competition (markets) or hierarchy (bureaucracies); and (c) the ultimate goal of this interaction is to define public policy processes and/or outcomes measured against some degree of common decision-making. Types of cross-sectoral collaboration that have these three attributes qualify as policy networks.

The primary goal of this chapter is to identify the causal mechanisms that maximize collaborative capacity within policy networks as defined above. Capacity is an overall and aggregate measure of cross-sectoral collaboration at the network level. Three sets of mechanisms will be elaborated as the main factors behind higher levels of NCC: structural, relational, and institutional.

Structural and relational mechanisms are network-level factors that contribute to higher levels of collaborative capacity. Institutional mechanisms refer to those environmental factors with an influence on intra-network interaction. Combinations of these factors produce different levels of network collaborative, which puts networks on a continuum or scale of collaboration. Previous research has highlighted the importance of treating networks as part of a continuum which encompasses sufficient diversity (Bressers, O'Toole, & Richardson, 1994; Rhodes & Marsh, 1992) and "identifying useful analytical touchstones that should enable researchers to differentiate various forms of governance" (Jordan et al., 2005, p. 478).

The Structural Mechanisms of Network Collaboration

Even though they are often perceived as fluid and malleable, policy networks presume certain structural mechanisms that encourage mutual exchange within a horizontal organizational structure. Networks do not have a fixed structure that is strictly defined. Instead of a rigid structure, networks are built upon linkages or bonds that connect actors within one framework of interaction, communication, and exchange. The looseness/flexibility of network structure is due to the intertwined nature of structure and agency at the network level (Marsh & Smith, 2000). Thus, structure is about the geometry of collaboration, referring to all those mechanisms that facilitate reciprocal and mutual exchange among network participants, and, therefore contribute to higher levels of collaborative capacity. Most of the previous studies define structure in terms of the alignment of the actors within the network. Therefore, the word "structure" is used to examine the position of actors within network structures based on intra-network elements such as links, nodes, centrality, density, and hierarchy (Provan & Kenis, 2008; Wasserman & Faust, 1994).

Previous studies do not directly refer to mechanisms of network collaboration as such. Instead, researchers focus on networks as organizations with specific constituting elements that bond network participants together. Among others, researchers discuss "intra-network exchange," "symbiotic relationship," "arrangements of interdependence," "shared community of views," "concerted co-ordination" (Bressers et al., 1994); "resource interdependence," "game-like interaction," "continuing interaction" (Rhodes, 1996); or "systemic co-ordination," "games about rule," "common purpose," "joint-working capacity," "exchange of resources" (Stoker, 1998); or "technical necessities" and "formal and informal institutions" of network governance (Raab, 2002). Rod Rhodes (1996) highlights some structural network features such as resource interdependence, game-like interaction, and continuing interaction as the main characteristics of network governance.

Unlike previous research, I argue that the elements mentioned above may not be present in all networks, and, therefore, should not be treated as necessary features or constituting components of policy networks. Considering the fluid nature of networks, it would be more appropriate to treat the above "network features" as "mechanisms," which are open to empirical investigation and are eventually used to assess and compare different degrees of network collaboration across policy settings and policy areas. For the sake of illustration and clarification, let's take the example of interdependence as an element of policy networks. Interdependence may not be present in all instances of network collaboration, and even if that is the case, interdependence is expected to show variations in terms of degree and form. A similar logic will be followed with other elements of policy networks listed above. This approach sits well within those accounts that call for a broader conceptualization and operationalization of policy networks in order to include diverse forms of network collaboration found in different institutional set-ups (Kjaer, 2011). The structural mechanisms that will be applied in this study are network features or components covered and emphasized in previous research and considered relevant to network definition applied in this study. These mechanisms summarized in Table 1 – namely (a) inclusiveness, (b) connectedness, (c) common decision-making, (d) interdependence, and (e) horizontal coordination – will be discussed briefly in the following paragraphs.

Inclusiveness: Network inclusiveness is about the breadth or scope of collaboration, referring to the range of actors involved in a cooperative project. Going back to the definition of policy networks provided in this study, policy networks involve cross-sectoral collaboration. Practically, this means that policy networks do not refer to multi-organization/inter-organizational/inter-institutional networks only

Table 1. Network Structural Capacity.

Structural Capacity	
Inclusiveness	Input-related mechanisms (broad, representative, cross-sectorial engagements).
Connectedness	Effective communication mechanisms.
Continuing interaction	Frequent communication mechanisms (frequent, regular interactions).
Face-to-face communication	Close communication mechanisms (direct, physical contacts).
Common decision-making	Decision-making mechanisms (vs. consultative and operational processes).
Interdependence	Mutual reliance mechanisms.
Resource pooling	Benefit sharing mechanisms (exchange of tangible and intangible resources).
Binding rules and regulations	Enforcement mechanisms (commonly agreed regularities, mutual understanding).
Horizontal coordination	Leveling mechanisms (horizontal alignment of actors).
Equal bargaining power	Equal bargaining mechanisms (mutual exchange of ideas regardless of organizational affiliation).
Efficient self-coordination	Self-organizing mechanisms (vs. lead agency management).

but to multi-sectoral/cross-sectoral networks that require the involvement of public, private, and voluntary actors in policy making. In contexts such as Turkey, networks with no cross-sectoral dynamics carry the risk of reproducing patterns of hierarchy and authority and, eventually, lose the essence of network collaboration. Here network collaboration essentially refers to a process where a wide range of actors from public, private, and voluntary sectors meet regularly and frequently in order to achieve consensual or mutually acceptable results with some measurable impact on policy making process and outcomes. Hence, webs of relations between public organizations only, such as platforms of inter-governmental collaboration, do not qualify as networks in this study. High levels of actor inclusiveness demonstrate that different sectors and organizations are recognized as legitimate actors in the policy making processes. An inclusive structure serves the purpose of representation from a wide range of policy sectors. The argument here is that policy networks with high collaborative capacity take the form of inclusive platforms that represent various types of stakeholders from the public, private, and voluntary sectors.

The concept of inclusiveness, which is essentially about the typology of actors, should not be conflated with network size, which is about the number of actors within a network, or network density, which is about the number of possible linkages/potential relationships among organizations participating in collaborative projects. Even though inclusiveness, size and density pertain to the input side of network policy making, they represent slightly different notions. For the purpose of this study, inclusiveness acquires particular importance accounting for the cross-sectoral aspect of network collaboration. Cross-sectoral network collaboration is critical in policy areas such as health, which are inherently inter-sectoral (Peters, Klijn, Stronks, & Harting, 2017).

Connectedness: Connectedness or inter-connectedness is one of the essential elements in network analysis. "The central argument of network research is that actors are embedded in networks of inter-connected social relationships that offer opportunities for and constraints on behavior" (Brass, Galaskiewicz, Greve, & Tsai, 2004, p. 795); meaning that networks are not about actors per se but about their connectedness. In this study, connectedness refers to those effective communication mechanisms that bond network participants together within a collaborative network structure. Connectedness consists of both continuing interaction and face-to-face communication, which are equally important in fostering NCC. In this study, continuing interaction refers to the frequency of communication among network participants. Previous literature emphasizes continuing interaction as a critical component in policy networks. Network participants are expected to build a recurrent or continuing relationship among each other. According to Rod Rhodes (1996, 2007), continuing interaction is one of the main attributes of governance networks. He argues that a continuous flow of communication between network members is "caused by the need to exchange resources and negotiate shared purposes" (Rhodes, 2007, p. 1246). Other following studies have also paid attention to the role of communication flow in a policy network. Communication ties are expected to maintain resource flows, reduce uncertainty, and fulfill roles (Rethemeyer & Hatmaker, 2007, p. 635), which are tasks necessary for network operation.

However, we cannot expect all policy networks to be characterized by frequent, smooth, and uninterrupted flows of communication. The degree and the impact of frequent communication on network effectiveness should be open to research. The argument here is that frequent communication is expected to strengthen collaboration among network participants. Face-to-face communication is another mechanism that contributes to connectedness, and eventually, collaborative capacity in policy networks. Face-to-face communication involves direct and physical communication, which is expected to be more effective that indirect communication via phone or internet. Previous research has shown that face-to-face communication makes network interaction more collaborative (Ansell & Gash, 2008). Apart from face-to-face communication, virtual channels of communication are becoming increasingly popular in contemporary policy making practices. Actually, both virtual and face-to-face communications are critical for network connectedness. Previous research suggests that "virtual and in person activities led to greater feelings of connectedness, and an ability of stakeholders to see and experience the opinions of a greater variety of community members" (Janssen & Helbig, 2018, p. 102). Nevertheless, for the purpose of this study face-to-face communication is particularly important as a channel of communication that facilitates knowledge exchange, mutual persuasion, and policy learning – features associated with policy networks. As stated previously "interpersonal communication is typically required to persuade someone of the importance of an issue or of a needed behavior change" (Moser & Dilling, 2007, p. 687).

Common Decision-making: There is extended debate in the existing literature concerning the impact of networks on policy outcomes or the extent to which networks can shape policies. However, understanding the link between policy networks and policy outcomes turns out to be a challenging task. According to Marsh and Smith (2000):

> [...] when a decision is made within a particular network, it is not simply the result of a rational assessment of available options ... but rather reflects past conflicts and the culture and values of decision makers. As such, networks do affect policy outcomes but not in a simple way. (p. 6)

The underlying assumption is that policy networks are expected to shape policy processes and outcomes through some degree of decision-making among network participants. Common decision-making is one of the trickiest elements in network analysis. Especially if one follows an institutionalist perspective, "a principal characteristic of these issue networks is that it is difficult to trace the locus of decision-making. The dependencies and power relations are diffuse" (Jordan & Schubert, 1992, p. 22). In addition, decision-making processes are complex, lengthy, and involved actors tend to change over time (Klijn, Steijn, & Edelenbos, 2010). Despite the diffused, lengthy, complex nature of decision-making, the definition of policy networks in this book assumes some degree of common decision-making in order to be able to distinguish policy networks from platforms that are essentially consultative or operational in nature and with minimal or almost no impact on policy outcomes.

Against this background, it becomes critical to scrutinize instances of common decision-making in every stage of policy making separately rather than only focusing on final policy outcomes. The argument put forward here is that policy collaboration at the stage of policy design and formulation is expected to involve more common decision-making among network participants compared to other stages of policy making such as agenda building (consultative nature), policy implementation (operational nature), or evaluation. Collaboration at the stage of policy implementation is most probably due to technical requisites rather than a product of genuine common decision-making, which is most probably the case in earlier stages of policy making (Bressers et al., 1994, p. 7). Even though the policy formulation stage is expected to involve more common decision-making, all policy stages involve some degree of common decision-making. For instance, if network collaboration takes place from agenda building to the policy evaluation stage of policy making, that network scores high in terms of common decision-making compared to another case that involves network collaboration only at the policy implementation stage. The argument here is that policy networks that facilitate common decision-making among network participants exhibit higher levels of NCC.

Interdependence: Previous studies have considered interdependence as a defining attribute of policy networks. In the literature, interdependence is defined strictly as network participants' reliance on each other in terms of financial resources. In this study, interdependence is conceived as a multi-faceted concept and is defined broadly in terms of those mutual reliance mechanisms that enable coordination among actors within network structure. Interdependence is built upon two main components: resource pooling and organizational rules. Resource pooling represents the financial or knowledge exchange side (resource interdependence), whereas organizational rules represent the job division or the organizational side (task interdependence). The argument here is that policy networks with collaborative capacity are platforms that facilitate an interdependent relationship among their participants built upon resource interdependence and organizational rules.

Resource interdependence is considered by many scholars to be the main feature of network structure (Park & Rethemeyer, 2012; Rhodes, 1996). In recent years, interdependence has grown due to the fact that "the boundaries between public, private and voluntary sectors became shifting and opaque" (Rhodes, 2007, p. 1246). Interdependence is observed particularly in policy environments where resources are scarce. Research has shown that resource interdependence among cross-sectoral organizations is primarily financial in nature but also takes the form of "staff, premises, information, legitimacy, and legal authority" (Lundin, 2007). For the purpose of this study, two broad categories of resource interdependence will be investigated: (1) material/financial and/or (2) knowledge-based interdependence (expertise or local knowledge). The presence of material and knowledge-based interdependence together, sums up to higher levels of interdependence among actors.

As indicated above, resource interdependence often entails financial interdependence, as that is the most commonly faced type of interdependence among network participants. Public policy in general, and social policy in particular, is characterized by dispersed costs and shared benefits. As a result, public policy costs and expenses are more prone to be shared by multiple actors. This could either mean that finances are shared by some organizations (system of dispersed or diffused costs) or that money financed by one organization/agency is used by some other organizations. The latter is usually the case in publicly funded projects where state agencies are the principal funders (governance networks can be solely publicly funded).

Knowledge-based interdependence is either about the continuous sharing of expertise or about sharing local area knowledge. Expertise is about formal and technical competences of actors involved in the network. Public agencies collaborate with private agencies, which possess technical knowledge in one specific area. Expertise could also be shared through network-level competences (Provan & Kenis, 2008), which is a more advanced version of knowledge-based resource interdependence. As the name indicates, "coordinating skills and task-specific competences" (Provan & Kenis, 2008, p. 240) are at the network level, rather than one or two organizations possessing a certain skill and being responsible for one task.

Interdependence on local area knowledge, on the other hand, is usually studied in the context of community-based services within the health policy sector. Community-based human service sub-networks are largely non-profit and voluntary, that is, interaction is not based on exchange of financial resources. In such cases, the tie that keeps community-based actors together is the "knowledge base that non-profit organizations have developed in a particular service area" (Alexander, Nank, & Stivers, 1999, p. 461). This type of "local knowledge" can include social sources of information such as information about the area where services are provided or information about social groups dwelling in that area. This kind of knowledge derives from the familiarity and legitimacy that the non-profit organizations should enjoy within the community in which they operate.[1] In this case, non-profit organizations use local knowledge as repository to build local-level networks, which are wide spread within the health policy area, especially in terms of providing mental health and psychosocial support services.

Overall, resource interdependence between different actors is considered to be a central factor for the emergence and development of policy networks (Huang & Provan, 2006). Moreover, research has shown that mutual resource dependence increases cooperation at the inter-organizational level (Levine & White, 1961; Van de Ven & Walker, 1984). Building upon these findings, resource interdependence is expected to have a positive effect on actors' capacity to collaborate with the purpose of policy making at the network level.

Apart from resource sharing, rules and regulations represent the organizational side of interdependence, which will be referred to as enforcement mechanisms here. In a way, what binds several actors together is task fulfillment regulated by commonly agreed upon rules. The closest concept to organizational rules is that of game-like interaction as described by Rhodes. According to Rhodes (2007),

---

[1]One instance of this type of network could be community-based non-profit/civil society organizations that provide services for people with mental illnesses or other children and family services (Huang & Provan, 2006).

intra-network interaction is "rooted in trust and regulated by rules of the game negotiated and agreed by network participants" (p. 1246). Rules here do not refer to a strict and fixed set of regulations, it is network participants who decide about the rules, which is more complicated than it seems. In a network there are no "rules of the game" but rather "games about rules" (Stoker, 1998). The underlying premise here is that network participants are rational actors, who can act strategically and adjust their behavior according to the constraints posed by the rules.

In more concrete terms, rules constrain the action of network participants through *ex ante* or *ex post* controls. *Ex ante* controls refer to administrative rules, guidelines, goals, or mandates agreed upon at the beginning of network collaboration. *Ex ante* controls, in a way, preclude non-compliant decisions or actions. *Ex post* controls, on the other hand, punish the acts of non-compliance to the terms and conditions of the agreement or contract. Networks do not always have clear goals, rules, or mandates that regulate the interactions among network members. Yet, many scholars have paid attention to the study of rules as an important dimension of network structure.

Previous research emphasizes that rules give policy networks stability. Network participants "interact in rather similar ways and reproduce more or less the same set of rules and resources" (Klijn, 1996, p. 101). Following this logic, rules are particularly useful in creating a collaborative structure that furthers the interaction between network participants by playing the same game over and over (Klijn, 1996, p. 100). "Clear and accepted conflict-regulating mechanisms promote cooperation and interactions" (Klijn, 2001, p. 160). This approach pays special attention to steering or management as critical for policy collaboration at the network level. Based largely on this perspective, the argument here is that various enforcement mechanisms that regulate relations among network participants contribute to higher levels of NCC.

Horizontal Coordination: Horizontal coordination represents an essential dimension of policy networks, which encapsulates those "leveling" mechanisms that balance the positions of different actors and make mutual exchange among them possible in practice. These mechanisms contribute to actor alignment within a horizontal structure of interaction. The proposition here is that flatter network structures perpetuate equal bargaining, adding to higher levels of NCC.

Power relations are an indispensable aspect of network analysis that cannot be ignored (van Waarden, 1992). Previous studies show that networks can be defined as "relatively stable horizontal articulation of interdependent, but operationally autonomous actors" (Sørensen & Torfing, 2005, p. 197). From a political or power perspective, policy networks are platforms that facilitate horizontal interaction between state and non-state actors. The premise here is that there might be power differences between network participants, yet, those differences can be leveled or balanced through equal bargaining mechanisms within the network structure. Critical decision-making serves as a litmus test for the presence of equal bargaining power among actors. It is during such moments that certain actors tend to dominate others. All in all, equal bargaining mechanisms allow actors to negotiate their position and ideas regardless of status, position, organizational affiliation, or type of decision-making, leading to higher levels of NCC.

Beyond the political/power dimension, horizontal coordination also has a managerial dimension. Network management is increasingly gaining importance especially with regard to performance-related issues in network analysis (Peters et al., 2017). In this context, the presence of efficient self-coordination (Scharpf & Mohr, 1994) through self-organizing mechanisms (Berardo & Scholz, 2010) or through joint information systems accessible by all network participants (Kapucu, 2006), gains particular importance. These mechanisms, either combined or separately, are expected to contribute to the horizontal coordination of the network, leading to higher levels of NCC.

Relational Mechanisms of Network Collaboration

Relational mechanisms refer to the nature of interaction within networks by paying particular attention to the ways in which network participants bond with each other. The existing literature largely acknowledges that network relations are organized by the principle of trust. Several studies within the domain of policy making and public management have found that trust among network participants serves as a mechanism that fosters collaboration at the network level (Agranoff & McGuire, 2001; Bardach, 1998; Fulda et al., 2012; Isett & Provan, 2005; Klijn et al., 2016; Lundin, 2007; McGuire, 2006; Peters et al., 2017; Provan & Kenis, 2008). As one of the most essential characteristics that distinguishes networks from markets and hierarchies, "[t]rust is essential for co-operative behaviour and, therefore, the existence of the network" (Sørensen & Torfing, 2007, p. 79). However, relatively scant effort has been directed toward empirically measuring the effect of trust on the collaborative capacity of policy networks. The aim of this study is to conceptualize and operationalize trust as a mechanism that fosters collaboration at the network level, which is a truly challenging task considering the multi-faceted and multi-level character of trust.

Trust is a truly interdisciplinary concept studied from various research perspectives ranging from philosophical, sociological, and psychological to economic, legal, and political science approaches. Furthermore, trust is one of the least tangible and intelligible concepts, not easily studied through quantifiable measures. The network perspective of trust focuses on the idea that collective action takes place in a situation of risk (Berardo, 2009). In other words, network participants engage in collective action despite the risk associated with the opportunistic behavior of other network participants. The risk of opportunistic behavior refers to the possible occurrence that other network participants will not work toward common goals but toward their particularistic interests. One of the main arguments in the literature is that trust emerges when network participants approach each other as partners who fulfill their own commitments and work toward common goals despite the risk factors associated with opportunistic behavior. For the purpose of this study, intra-network trust is manifested at both the inter-personal and inter-organizational levels. Different levels and forms of trust are summarized in Table 2 and explained in a more detailed fashion in the following paragraphs.

Previous studies suggest that trust within networks can be measured at the inter-personal level in the form of inter-personal credibility. Inter-personal level

Table 2. Network Relational Capacity.

Relational Capacity			
Inter-personal Level Trust			
Credibility, loyalty, informal relations, social ties, family-like atmosphere, friendliness...			
Inter-organizational Level Trust			
(a) Reputation-based form of trust Trust is present from the beginning of network collaboration. Organization's status, reputation, credibility, and legitimacy.			
(b) Performance-based form of trust Trust evolves during the process of network collaboration. Willingness to cooperate, solidarity, team work, synergy.			
Low..High			
Willingness to cooperate Lingering organizational differences.	*Solidarity* Agreeing on shared goals. Some degree of productiveness.	*Team work* Splitting up tasks and responsibilities. Productive group work.	*Synergy* Motivating work environment. Highly productive group work.

trust is essentially about trust between individuals who represent organizations because, in reality, "it is not an organization that trusts, but rather the individuals who constitute it" (Janowicz & Noorderhaven, 2006, p. 265). A useful approach is one provided by Curral and Judge (1995), who define inter-organizational trust as the individual's behavioral reliance on another person under a condition of risk. According to this study, which was conducted in the United States, inter-organizational trust can best be measured at the individual level, as "trust between the individuals who provide the linking mechanism across organizational boundaries, namely, boundary role persons" (Curral & Judge, 1995, pp. 151–152). "Trust is formed by individuals (within certain organizations in the network) in their interactions with other individuals (in other organizations)" (Klijn et al., 2016, p. 117). Hence, network level trust can be described as a combination of inter-personal and inter-organizational elements of trust, which will be further elaborated below.

Inter-personal level trust: Inter-personal level relations often arise in the absence of formal rules and regulations, and therefore, can be perceived as a proxy for informal relations. There seems to be a perception that the absence of formal rules and regulations implies the presence of inter-personal trust, as there is no need for external constraints to buttress trust between individuals. The reasoning behind this approach is that formal rules check against the risks coming from an untrustworthy organization or individual. Previous studies have considered informal agreements between organizations as a measure of trust (Curral & Judge, 1995) and, moreover, have found that rising levels of informality over time lead to increased levels of trust (Gulati, 1995). Therefore, an understanding that "informality breeds trust" (Gulati, 1995) is already present in the literature. This perspective on trust would be applicable in cases where intra-network relations involve some degree of informality through strong inter-personal relations or in the presence of spoken rules instead of written rules of agreement or contract enforcement.

For the sake of clarification, the argument put forward here does not advocate informal relations as intrinsically better or superior compared to formal relations within a policy network. Network relations do not pose a dilemma of trade-off between informality and formality. The rise of informal ties does not necessarily imply diminishing formal, that is, contractual ties. In practice, network relationships involve a mix of formal and informal ties, with contribute to the development of trust within networks in a variety of institutional configurations. Previous research on intra-organizational culture in Turkey has shown that there is a close connection between trust and informal relations. Successful leaders are expected to be caring, responsive, and close to their employees as well as maintain a "family-like atmosphere" within the organization (Fikret Paşa, Kabasakal, & Bodur, 2001). Hence, in the Turkish context, inter-personal relations in the form of credibility, loyalty, social ties, family-like atmosphere, or friendliness, should be taken in account in the examination of trust different levels of analysis.

Inter-organizational level trust: Organization studies within the field of management pay particular attention to trust at the inter-organizational level, which is crucial to understand trust in network analysis. Inter-organizational level trust could be a function of an organization's reputation and status but could also be a task-based form of trust that takes the form of solidarity, team work, or synergy. In the former case, network participants display a trusting behavior early in the process of network collaboration in a more automatic fashion, whereas in the latter case, trust is expected to evolve during the process of collaboration depending upon several criteria of task performance and commitment.

Reputation is about the credibility that an organization enjoys within its own sector. Organizational attributes such as reputation or legitimacy are crucial for the analysis of inter-organizational trust (Ganesan & Hess, 1997; Van de Ven & Ring, 2006). This dimension of trust is a "strategic-level trust," which is:

> crucially important in partner selection and alliance formation stages of collaboration, thus finding manifestation primarily in the collaborative policies of the firm and the collaborative arrangements of the particular alliances. (Janowicz & Noorderhaven, 2006, p. 273)

Reputation-based forms of trust are more likely to emerge in strategic partnerships or in recurring business-oriented networks where there is a certain amount of trust accumulated through previous work experience. In such cases, trust is present from the beginning of the collaborative process and emerges in more or less automatic fashion. This argument, however, requires some qualification. In reality, partner selection and alliance formation stages of collaboration, mentioned above, do not always reveal much about the sentiment of trust in the long run. Stated differently, the emergence of trust in early stages of network collaboration does not guarantee its persistence throughout the process of network collaboration. Collaboration could start with a trust vacuum and develop into a very good working relationship, or, the very opposite could be the case. So, the way relations evolve during the process of network collaboration matters as well.

Task-oriented forms of trust, on the other hand, do not emerge automatically. They are a function of processes of collaboration among network participants depending on their contribution and commitment to overall network goals. This conceptualization of trust is similar to James Coleman's (1988) definition of social capital – considered as the network-based approach to social capital. Coleman (1988) highlights that "like other forms of capital, social capital is productive, making possible the achievement of certain ends that in its absence would not be possible" (p. 98). Network level social capital can be defined in terms of "network productiveness" or "network goal achievement." Following this logic, one way to define social capital is the enhancement of goal achievement through social interaction at the network level. Drawing a parallel to social capital, a task-oriented form of trust can be conceptualized as the willingness of network participants to participate in collaborative policy making and contribute to overall goal achievement. This definition implies that network participants are competent enough to offer a valuable contribution to a network's overall productiveness and goal achievement. A similar operationalization of trust is provided by Klijn et al. (2016), where a significant relationship is built between network level trust and network performance.

In order to fully comprehend the notion of trust, or trust-building as a process, one should investigate the way trust evolves over time. In some cases, some exchange prior to network formation among stakeholders is necessary to build trust. In some other cases, trust among network participants is already there, however, that trust strengthens or weakens during the process of collaboration. Overall, trust is expected to increase over time, building up to higher levels of network collaboration. To illustrate this point, high levels of trust-based interaction can even be perceived as an advanced form of network collaboration. This situation is best described by integration theories of network governance which defend the idea that:

> [o]ver time, governance networks develop their own logic of appropriateness, which is often influenced by isomorphic pressures .... The network actors become normatively and cognitively integrated through the construction of solidarity and common identities and frames of reference. (Sørensen & Torfing, 2007, p. 19)

Following this logic, this study builds a scale of trust, which consists of consecutive steps of trust-building, namely – (a) willingness to cooperate against diverging interests, goals, and strategies; (b) goal convergence or agreement on shared goals manifested in the form of solidarity; (c) team work (productiveness) through task or responsibility sharing; and (d) synergetic relationship (innovation) or highly productive team work leading to mutual learning, knowledge exchange, and innovation. Each of these steps serves as a proxy for different levels of trust.

Willingness to cooperate and goal convergence represent less developed forms of trust at the network level. Willingness to cooperate represents the minimum possible level of trust that brings various actors together. Goal convergence is a critical element that bonds network participants from the early stages of network collaboration. Previous studies have found that diverging goals and objectives may hamper cooperation (O'Toole, 2003). Moreover, goal congruence promotes joint action and policy collaboration if bolstered by mutual trust between organizations (Lundin, 2007). Provan and Kenis (2008) argue that goal-directed networks, which have a specific purpose and mandate, are essential mechanisms for achieving multi-organizational outcomes (p. 231). Other studies have highlighted goal consensus as a mechanism that regulates network level interaction. In this sense, goal consensus does not require all network participants to have the same goals and instead is about agreeing on broad network level goals. For the purpose of this study, what really matters is the degree to which network participants agree on a set of common goals, despite differing preferences, interests, and motivations, which are necessary to preclude contentious competition and conflict among network participants. However, at this stage one cannot talk about a fully developed form of trust or a very cohesive policy network. This type of trust is witnessed in the so-called American variant of issue networks (Bressers et al., 1994, p. 12), which are relatively less cohesive networks.

Team work and synergetic relations reflect more developed forms of trust leading to higher levels of network exchange, productiveness, and performance. Team work is characterized by the effective division of labor, where each network participant contributes toward common goals in a specific way. At the same time, network participants are well-connected to each other through high levels of information exchange. This type of network resembles the dense and tightly connected groups, described by Coleman in his study (1988), which are likely to develop trust among their participants. Here, team work represents medium levels of trust and is expected to be observed in well-connected and cohesive policy networks. Finally, a synergetic relationship refers to separate contributions that mutually reinforce each other toward commonly shared goals. These types of interaction are characterized by high levels of trust which translate into positive synergy among network participants leading to high levels of network performance.

Institutional Mechanisms of Network Collaboration

The study of internal mechanisms of network collaboration has been extensively covered in the literature, particularly within the NGS. Yet, the study of external factors shaping network dynamics, such as the broader political and economic institutions, remains underdeveloped. Network governance approaches do not emphasize the role of the broader institutional framework where the policy networks are situated and immersed. According to these approaches, ideal type policy networks are often conceived as "autonomous" and "self-regulating" entities (Rhodes, 1996, 1997). Such a definition gives rise to the misperception that networks are policy instruments isolated from their surrounding political environment. This could hold true in those political environments which are favorable to the network logic and pattern of governance. In such cases, the broader political environment within which networks come into being is taken for granted.

The study of the surrounding institutions helps researchers look at policy networks as entities that operate within a larger system. Actually, no policy making environment can illustrate power relations more vividly than policy networks, which are found at the intersection of various policy preferences, interests, and power games. Policy networks consist of a variety of actors, who presumably have some degree of power and "interact through negotiations that involve bargaining, deliberation and intensive power struggles" (Sørensen & Torfing, 2005, p. 197). Based on this assumption, policy networks are often shaped by different external factors pertaining to the surrounding political and economic environment. In this way, policy networks cannot be exempted from either the political and economic interests or from the power relations behind formal policy networks. Networks can even be defined as platforms where "different actors struggle with each other, create opportunities for joint decisions, forge political compromises and coordinate concrete actions" (Sørensen & Torfing, 2007, p. 27).

Clearly, policy networks reflect different power relations among actors in the broader political and economic institutional environment. However, the ways in which these political and economic institutions affect policy networks (as institutions in their own right) is not clearly explained in the literature. Neo-institutionalist approaches are particularly useful to understand network embeddedness within the broader institutional environment (Blom-Hansen, 1997; Bogason & Toonen, 1998; Lowndes, 2001; Lowndes & Roberts, 2013; Toonen, 1998). The neo-intuitionalist approach expands the scope of network analysis by focusing on actors, relations, and interests external to policy networks rather than focusing exclusively on networks as closed organizations. The assumption here is that policy networks are not isolated entities; on the contrary, they are embedded in the broader institutional environment that surrounds them. Drawing from this approach, the institutionalization of policy networks becomes a function of the surrounding political and economic institutions external to network structure. In the same vein, institutional mechanisms refer to factors external to network structure with a power to influence intra-network collaboration. This argument is closely linked to the notion of "institutional embeddedness," that is, the degree to which policy networks are immersed in the surrounding political and economic environment.

A mix of factors are investigated in this study to gauge institutionalization of policy networks through (a) prevailing discourses concerning the policy area under investigation (media discourses, EU/WHO discourses, and pre-election discourses); (b) prominent political leaders or high-level state officials within the policy area under investigation; (c) political or business-based alignments within the policy area under investigation (alliances or coalitions among elites involved in policy making); and (d) the presence of legislation or formal institutions related to the policy area (see Table 3). First, ideas and discourses are critical in shaping the political agenda. For instance, media discourses often shape policy making by framing, shifting, or legitimizing political and policy agenda. Thus, they are influential in the legitimization/legitimation and persistence of certain policy networks. Second, lead political actors with an impact on decision-making and

Table 3. Network Institutional Capacity.

Institutional Capacity			
Low..			...............High
Presence of prevailing discourses in the policy sub-area	Presence of prominent political leaders or state officials	Existing political coalitions and/ or business-based alliances	Presence of legislation and formal institutions in the policy sub-area

high-level state officials initiate policies (create new institutions or political agendas) or introduce policy changes (transforming existing institutions).[2] In some political contexts, prominent politicians and state officials, in spite of being outside the formal policy network, play an extremely important role in the formation and maintenance of policy networks. Third, political coalitions or business-based alliances are existing webs of relations which are not often in the public eye but are powerful enough to influence policy networks through implicit power relations. In that sense, it is possible to consider them as "background actors" (Bressers et al., 1994), or actors who shape intra-network interaction through political or financial support. Finally, highly institutionalized networks operate within a legal and formal institutional framework.

Based on the premises of the neo-institutionalist approach, the institutional resilience of policy networks is closely linked to prevailing discourses/ideas, prominent political leaders/high-level state officials, the presence of business alliances/political coalitions, and the presence of legal and institutional frameworks in the respective policy area. The argument here is that institutional resilience does contribute to network persistence or sustainability, and, at the same time, greater collaborative capacity at the network level.

Conclusion

Despite becoming a widespread mode of governance, particularly in the advanced industrialized countries, an approach for the study of policy networks outside the context of advanced democracies is largely missing in the literature. Asserting the value of universality to certain concepts, which are specific to political environments found in the advanced democracies, weakens not only the comparative dimension but also the overall plausibility of those concepts. This chapter contends that the lack of a comparative framework is the root problem in current debates on policy networks, in which researchers find themselves either studying ideal cases, often perceived as desirable cases of governance, or less than ideal cases without any theoretical or policy implications. These latter cases constitute unique and often unrelated practices that cannot be assessed in accordance with a standard criteria of comparison.

[2]Institutional Entrepreneurship literature offers a wide variety of studies on lead actors.

This chapter is an attempt to overcome this epistemological challenge by constructing an integrated framework that enables comparison across different country cases and policy settings at the sub-national and sub-sectoral levels. The framework suggested here takes into account both contextual conditions that give rise to network collaboration in the first place as well as causal mechanisms that strengthen network collaboration once they are formed. The underlying assumption here is that:

> credible causal explanation can occur if and only if researchers are attentive to the interaction between causal mechanisms and context, regardless of whether the methods employed are small-sample, formal, statistical, or interpretive. (Falleti & Lynch, 2009, p. 1)

Assuming that contextual conditions depend upon temporal and spatial factors peculiar to the case under investigation (Chapter 3 of this book), this chapter focuses exclusively on the causal mechanisms that strengthen network collaboration. The causal mechanisms identified in this chapter can be aggregated at the network level to construct the composite index of NCC, which has been utilized in the analysis of policy networks within the Turkish health sector (Chapter 4 of this book).

The aim here is to build an integrated framework that synthesizes causal mechanisms, namely structural, relational, and institutional factors which add up to overall network collaborative capacity as a measurement. These mechanisms are neither mutually exclusive nor individually adequate to explain network dynamics. In this study, structural, relational, and institutional factors are treated as equally important aspects of network collaboration, which should be investigated within one integrated framework. These factors, along with their constituting elements, contribute toward a better understanding of NCC at the conceptual level. It should be noted here that network capacity – unlike network performance that is more domain specific, thematic, and evaluative – is more aggregate, cumulative, and indicative of the overall ability of public, private, and voluntary organizations to collaborate. Therefore, practically, structural, relational, and institutional factors serve as blueprint for organizing efforts that amount to higher levels of NCC in policy making processes.

The framework introduced here integrates factors that foster collaborative capacity of policy networks drawing primarily from the existing discussions the literature but also taking into account the network definition presented in this study. Technically, a measure of NCC should integrate all those components/elements associated with a concept or phenomenon to be studied. At the same time, the framework should be as neutral and parsimonious as possible in order to be applicable and transferrable across cases. As Lynn, Heinrich, and Hill (2000) have pointed out:

> Theory-based empirical research should seek to identify the most parsimonious model for estimating key causal relationships that can be generalized beyond the specific context of analysis .... Furthermore many possible causal explanations might be ruled out in particular research contexts on the basis of a priori reasoning or on the basis of well-designed empirical research. (p. 246)

When it comes to application, causal mechanisms are very much contingent upon the context under investigation. For instance, the same mechanisms can be operationalized differently, depending upon contextual conditions. This means that some of the explanations of the framework introduced here may be ruled out, whereas some others may become more prominent depending upon the context of the empirical research.

Ultimately, the suggested framework is expected to add comparative value to the concept of policy networks by facilitating comparative network analysis across country cases going beyond the camp of advanced industrialized economies with an established tradition in network collaboration, as well as across policy sectors and sub-sectors at the sub-national level. The latter are critical to empirically substantiate arguments on network collaboration as well as add explanatory value to policy networks as fundamental concepts in public administration, policy studies, and political science disciplines through detailed accounts of network structure, relations, and institutionalization. Studying networks at the sectoral and sub-sectoral levels accounts for those intricacies often neglected in network analysis. As Rhodes and Marsh (1992) have noted "cross-national studies cannot simply assume that national variations are significant. Sectoral variations may be more important and, in consequence, it is necessary to disaggregate and explore sub-sectoral variations" (p. 203). Actually, it has been shown that "the structure and membership of sub sectoral policy networks may substantially overlap with, or be quite distinct from, each other" (Rayner, Howlett, Wilson, Cashore, & Hoberg, 2001, p. 320).

Chapter 3

Tracing Origins: The Context of Network Formation in a Least Likely Policy Environment

Abstract

This chapter investigates the origins of cross-sectoral collaboration by exploring when and why policy networks form within the Turkish health sector – a least likely case for network formation. The analysis presented here draws on information collected from a number of official documents, semi-structured interviews with professional experts, and two multi-stakeholder meetings. Timewise, networks entered the policy jargon during the introduction of the Health Transformation Program in 2003. Yet, the years between 2011 and 2015 were ground-breaking in producing concrete cross-sectoral collaborative instruments of policy making. The findings of the analysis reveal that policy networks form as a result of central government's choice to devolve responsibility and expand the policy space with new issues and actors. Moreover, policy networks emerge not only during the times of policy change which has a reactionary, abrupt, and nature but also during the times of policy stability and legitimacy. These contextual factors are crucial in maintaining an atmosphere of trust among stakeholders, particularly between state and non-state actors. The refugee crisis and spreading securitization discourse in the post-2015 period explain the shifting policy and political agenda leading to public sector retrenchment from cross-sectoral projects within the field of health. This chapter intends to contribute to the literature of comparative public policy by examining the link between policy networks and policy change in addition to adding to the debates on network governance by exploring the processes of network formation. Finally, this chapter contributes to Turkish studies by examining the process of network formation within the Turkish health sector.

Keywords: Health system; network formation; policy legitimacy; policy networks; policy stability; Turkey

Network Policy Making within the Turkish Health Sector: Becoming Collaborative, 41–62

doi:10.1108/978-1-83867-094-820201004

> Thinking in terms of policy networks makes us see them everywhere. It can disguise the fact that in at least some instances network collaboration is not an inevitable course of action for modern government, but a choice. (Bresser, 2009, p. 124)

As discussed in the previous chapters, the last three decades have seen a proliferation of the studies on networks as instruments of policy making based on the logic of collaboration among actors from the public, private, and voluntary sectors. While researchers have made significant advances on study of network structure as well as the process and consequences of network collaboration, the first stages of network formation have remained unexplored. The emergence of policy networks has often been explained by the shift from hierarchical and centralized government toward collaborative and shared modes of governance in advanced democracies. In this context, policy networks refer to new governing entities autonomous from the state (Rhodes, 1997). However, it would not be realistic to expect a substantial transformation in governance patterns across all policy settings without clear empirical evidence (Kjaer, 2011). Similarly, it would be inaccurate to approach the emergence of policy networks as an inevitable and uniform process that takes place in all modern governments (Bressers, 2009). Neglecting variation in network formation is a problem, particularly in those contexts where a substantial shift toward shared modes of governance has not yet taken place and the involvement of non-state actors into policy making processes through networks is the exception rather than the rule. Consequently, the question naturally arises of when and why do policy networks emerge in these specific policy settings?

Considering this gap in the literature, this chapter aims to understand the conditions under which policy networks emerge within the Turkish policy space, a least favorable case for the emergence of cross-sectoral collaboration due to its past record of centralized policy making and the executive being primarily responsible for orchestrating the entire process of policy making from agenda building to policy evaluation stage in the form of an uninterrupted bureaucratic cycle shaped by inertia and hierarchy. In other words, the goal of this chapter is to reveal those factors that lead to the disruption of the bureaucratic cycle of policy making. To this end, the formation stage of policy networks within three health policy sub-areas (i.e., public health development, healthcare construction, and health tourism) will be examined. Hence, this chapter aims at understanding the formation of policy networks within the Turkish health sector as innovative policy instruments that involve cross-sectoral collaboration with an impact on policy making processes and/or outcomes. Two specific questions will be addressed in this section: (a) When did networks of collaboration emerge? and (b) What factors led to the emergence of cross-sectoral collaboration in the form of policy networks? Even though asked separately, these two questions reflect the very origins of network formation.

A retrospective policy analysis is necessary to understand how actors from different organizations get involved in relatively lengthy and costly processes of cross-sectoral collaboration initially. The analysis of health policies in Turkey begins with the establishment of the Ministry of Health and Social Affairs (MHSA) as the main authority in the public health system in Turkey. However, the focus is put on more recent political and institutional developments, with an emphasis on the post-2003 period which is the starting point of the Health Transformation Programme (HTP). Policy analysis in this chapter is substantiated by information gathered from semi-structured interviews with representatives from the public, private, and voluntary sector organizations involved in cross-sectoral collaboration within the health sector in Turkey, including multi-stakeholder meetings, several governmental documents, and secondary sources.

This chapter is divided into three consecutive sub-sections. The first section is a brief account of the policy making patterns within the health sector in Turkey from the establishment of MHSA up to year 2003, a period where policy networks as concrete instruments with an impact on policy making are completely missing. The second section traces the post-2003 period by highlighting three stages of distinct policy making within the Turkish health policy space. Here, particular emphasis is placed on the 2011–2015 years interval as a critical or pivotal juncture of policy network formation within the Turkish health sector. The chapter ends with some concluding remarks on the nature of network formation in Turkey and the implications for the broader literature.

Network Collaboration in Turkey: A Missing Policy Tradition

This section is not an exhaustive overview of all health policy reforms in Turkey, but rather a retrospective account of how health policies have been made over the years by covering five decades of centralized policy making up to 2003. The aim of this analysis is to understand who the main decision-makers or players in the system are and how they make their policy choices, rather than analyze how available policy choices affect the health of individual citizens. Hence, this chapter aims to examine the governance side of health policy. Over time, health policies in Turkey have traditionally been centrally planned and financed with the officials working in the Ministry of Health (MoH) holding the most influential positions in decision-making. Therefore, concerning policy making patterns, Turkey represents a typical case of hierarchical, bureaucratic decision-making with the government holding a clear monopoly and private and voluntary actors having no or minimal impact on policy processes.

Two main early developments defined the central government. The Ministry of Health and Social Affairs (MHOSA)[1] became the main responsible entity for planning and providing necessary health services. First, in 1954 health services in the provinces were all placed under the authority of the MHOSA which took over the former role of the municipalities (Atun et al., 2013). Secondly, the 1961 Law on the Socialization of Health Services promoted an integrated health scheme and again was managed by MHOSA as "the largest health service provider" (Aktulay, 1996, p. 14). Since the 1960s, the main actors in health policy

[1]The former name of the Ministry of Health in Turkey used until 1983. https://www.turkcebilgi.com/sa%C4%9Fl%C4%B1k_bakanl%C4%B1%C4%9F%C4%B1.

making have been the MoH, the State Planning Organization (SPO), the Grand National Assembly (GNA), and the Constitutional Court (see Savaş, Karahan, & Saka, 2002). The MoH has been primarily responsible for setting policy objectives, implementing strategic plans, and administering healthcare services, with some degree of authority over strategic planning. The MoH, a very centralized organization, has been the major player within the health system in terms of planning, implementation, and monitoring. The SPO, directly accountable to the office of the Prime Minister, has been primarily responsible for strategic planning including large-scale investments within the health sector. Strategic plans published by the SPO as well as other legislative arrangement have been approved by the GNA. Finally, the Constitutional Court has been responsible for ensuring the conformity of laws and legislation on health-related issues with the constitution. The Higher Education Council was formally granted a policy making function within the health system after 1981, yet, in practice, this institution has had no impact on planning and other policy making processes other than consultation (see Savaş et al., 2002). Even though the health system has for a long time been highly centralized, the aforementioned institutions have not been involved in common decision-making, and as a result, health policy making has been quite fragmented. For example, SPO strategic plans have not always translated into policy programs implemented by the MoH, and the legislation passed in the GNA has often been annulled by the Constitutional Court.

Centralization of the health system left no room for private, voluntary actors, or even public actors at the local level to contribute to policy making processes. Existing research shows that "between 1976 and 1983 the share of the private sector within total investment in both education and health [as two main public policy sectors] rarely exceeded ten percent" (Boratav, Yeldan, & Köse, 2000, p. 29). Many reforms were undertaken by consecutive governments to strengthen the role of the private sector in health service delivery and eventually decrease the burden of the state service providers. The idea of reform was introduced as early as the 1980s with the formulation of two legal provisions. First, "in the 1982 Constitution the state was defined as regulator of, but not responsible for healthcare services, which marked a shift in comprehension of the social state in Turkey" (Kartal, 2009, p. 36). Secondly:

> the fifth Five-Year Development Plan (Devlet Planlama Teşkilatı Müsteşarlığı, 1984) listed the fundamental principles of national health policy as follows: incentivizing private health institutions; the liberalization of the cost of services provided by those facilities; outsourcing of the public service provision. (Kartal, 2009, p. 36)

Hitherto, these legal provisions were not followed by concrete policy arrangements and did not bring any substantial changes in the role and responsibilities of existing actors as well as policy making patterns. The attempts to restrict the role of the state and liberalize the health system in general through a Basic Law on Health Care Services (Official Gazette No. 3359, 1987) prescribing a narrower role for the MoH, were hampered by a Constitutional Court ruling in 1987

(Yasar, 2011). Therefore, a substantial change in terms of the logic and instruments of policy making could not be introduced.

The idea of reform was restated more strongly in the 1990s consisting mainly of liberalization incentives put forward by the World Bank (WB) as the leading actor pushing for healthcare reforms all over the world. Due to the active involvement of WB, domestic health system restructuring became a global trend during this period. Turkey and the WB cooperated on different healthcare components in the early 1990s (Kahveci & Meads, 2008; Savaş et al., 2002). Turkey signed Health Transition Project-Loan Agreements with the WB which were followed by concrete steps in the direction of marketization. During these years the private sector was emerging as a new stakeholder with an increasing market share, yet no power to shape policy making processes. As recorded by Boratav et al.:

> From 1994 onwards, thanks to the generous incentives extended to private investors in education and health, entrepreneurs started to move into health and education at a significant rate, and the private sector's share in these sectors reached the 50 percent benchmark by 1996–97. (2000, p. 30)

The liberalization reforms carried out in the 1990s were at best limited, and failed to bring any substantial change to the governance of health policy. At the outset, these reforms were limited by definition. Liberalization was understood at that time as marketization or privatization of service delivery. However, a full-fledged reform package that would bring a complete restructuring of the health system both in term of policy design and implementation was lacking. In other words, health reforms in Turkey aimed at expanding the market forces rather than at expanding the policy space within the health system. Despite the attempts to incorporate the private sector in healthcare service provision, no major transformations that would facilitate the involvement of private actors into the decision-making processes were achieved during the 1980s and 1990s. In addition, reforms were limited by implementation. Despite many privatization reforms, the central and local governments had no capacity to regulate or even formally supervise the private sector. Institutional arrangements that enable regular communication and interaction between public and private actors were practically lacking. This vacuum in coordination led to huge tax leakages and inefficiencies in the health system. During this time, "the private health and life insurance sectors [were] characterized by cases of irregularities, high lapses, and unaccounted policy cancellations" (Boratav et al., 2000, p. 31). The private sector operated in a clientelistic and opportunistic fashion which hindered its own growth in the long run. As a result of the liberalization reforms carried out in the 1990s, the private sector turned into another "Gordian knot" rather than a reliable partner expected to contribute to the overhaul of a malfunctioning health system.

The root causes of the enduring and complicated problems within the Turkish health system can be traced to system-level factors including the reluctance of the consecutive governments to alter the policy making patterns and expand the health policy space. Despite the incentives to reform the health system, the policy making processes were stuck within a bureaucratic cycle which was inherently malfunctioning. There were two main handicaps in the existing policy making model within the health system in Turkey. The first handicap was a complete reliance on state planning and funding, despite low levels of state capacity to maintain an effectively functioning health system. At the system level, state funding could no longer be sustained, especially after the introduction of liberal policies to the Turkish economy in the 1980s. Structural adjustment of the 1980s led to financial cuts particularly in social policy sectors (i.e., health care and education). Eventually, Turkey's health sector entered a crisis phase in the 1990s. According to data provided by the OECD, the spending ratio of health care to gross domestic product (GDP) in 1997 was as low as 4.0 percent. This is a drastically low figure when compared to median OECD countries at 7.5 percent. In the same year Turkey scored the lowest per capita health spending ($260 per person) among 29 OECD countries compared to generous spenders such as the US ($3,925 per person) and the OECD median ($1,728 per person). Accordingly, the state lacked the financial means necessary to meet the healthcare challenges in Turkey.

Another weakness of health policy making in Turkey had to do with the minimal contribution of non-state actors which extensively operated in a chaotic environment without clear rules and regulations and completely distant from policy making processes. Despite many attempts to involve the private sector in healthcare service provision, no major transformations of the system were achieved during the 1990s. The incentives given to private investors in the 1990s were handled in a clientelistic and opportunistic fashion that hindered the growth of the private sector itself without generating any financial resources for the healthcare system in general. As a result, private sector actors never became capable enough to get involved in health policy making through collaborative relations with other public actors. The combination of these two system-level shortcomings (i.e., weak state capacity and lack of an institutional framework facilitating cooperation between state and non-state actors) has had detrimental effects on the healthcare system in Turkey over the years.

Overall, government institutions with the power to shape policy making lacked the financial, technical and managerial resources necessary to meet healthcare challenges in Turkey. On top of it, consecutive governments lacked the willingness to engage in collaborative policy making with other policy stakeholders to ameliorate the situation. This highly centralized and fragmented bureaucratic cycle turned into a vicious cycle that was pushing the healthcare system toward collapse. Contextual factors made this picture even more complicated. Among others, the instability of the Turkish political environment, especially in the 1990s, hampered the installation of serious bureaucratic and policy reforms within the health policy area. The 1990s are defined as a period of "extreme multipartisim with no dominant party" (Sayari & Esmer, 2002, p. 22). In the 1990s Turkey was led by coalition parties that did not share similar programs. Ironically, parties with similar programs and ideological positions were deliberately prevented from forming coalition governments due to the animosity and rivalry between their leaders (Sayari & Esmer, 2002, p. 29). Coalition governments, composed of ideologically distant political parties, lacked any clear position on health policy as well as other policies. In addition, the debates taking place in the Turkish GNA were continually characterized by a stalemate.

Up until the 2000s, Turkey can be characterized as an under-achiever or weak performer in the governance of health policies. Turkey's health system was virtually moving toward breakdown, a point where the system would not be able to meet the demands of the employers, employees, and patients. Since 2003, the Turkish health sector has undergone major reforms which were initiated by the adoption of the HTP by the "MoH" in 2003.[2] The year 2003 can be perceived as a critical juncture mainly due to the changes introduced within the health policy area. The following section traces policies introduced in the aftermath of 2003 under the HTP reform umbrella with the purpose of understanding the changing patterns of policy making.

The Origins of Collaboration: When and Why Did Policy Networks Emerge?

The objective of this section is to explore the conditions under which policy networks emerged within the Turkish health sector. Three-year intervals can be distinguished here, namely, 2003–2011, 2011–2015, and 2015 to the present. Each interval corresponds to periods where networks served as (a) an emerging policy frame/rhetoric, (b) as policy instruments utilized in cross-sectoral projects, and (c) as suspended projects due to changing political and policy priorities. In other words, this section aims at assessing the cycle of the rise and fall of network policy making by focusing on the years after the introduction of the HTP reforms in Turkey, when a new way of thinking about health governance was gradually yet steadily being developed within the public administration preceding the formation of policy networks during the 2011–2015 period.

Networks as a New Way of Thinking within Public Administration (2003–2011)

As discussed above, prior to 2003 the Turkish health system was not only going through a crisis period, it was immersed in a vicious cycle of policy making. Thus, immediate action was necessary both in terms of policy content and policy making patterns. It was not until the implementation of the HTP (2003) that the ideas of systemic change were brought into the political agenda and translated into concrete health policy goals and directives. The goal of this program was not to reform but transform the healthcare system. Therefore, it is possible to talk about the reconfiguration of the healthcare system as a whole. Turkey is one of the few countries that has implemented "broad multifaceted health system reforms" in an attempt to "develop their own reform model" (Bossert, 2012, p. 9).[3] HTP included

---

[2]See Atun et al. (2013), Ökem and Çakar (2015), and Yasar (2011) for a detailed account on HTP in Turkey.

[3]In his research Bossert lists other countries including Chile, China, Colombia, Ghana, Taiwan, and some Eastern European states.

several components with the power of transformative change such as increasing the MoH's capacity for stewardship, introducing universal health insurance, reorganizing health service delivery with particular attention given to family medicine and primary healthcare services, developing human resources and introducing a national health information system, increasing the involvement of municipalities, universities, professional organizations, private firms, and new specialized agencies responsible for education, scientific research, and management particularly in the field of pharmaceuticals and medical devices, promoting cross-border health services, and mobilizing stakeholders to engage in cross-sectoral collaboration (Yasar, 2011a).

Relatively few studies analyze the broad systemic changes associated with the reconfiguration of the healthcare system in Turkey, particularly the respective policy instruments and actors involved in policy making processes. On one hand, there is a tendency to focus on the consequences of the "liberal reforms" introduced in the post-2003 period (Ataay, 2008). On the other hand, there is a tendency to interpret reforms in light of a larger wave of marketization and privatization which began in Turkey in the 1980s (Kartal, 2009). Stating that the health system is moving in the direction of marketization is a misleading oversimplification. This conclusion is obtained as a result of a linear logic-based analysis in which healthcare can move either in the direction of state-controlled or in the direction of market-controlled policy making. Following this logic, policy making is a zero-sum game. It is either the state or market interests that define the health status of citizens. Another problem with this type of analysis is that it misses numerous details and intricacies concerning various actor constellations and policy making processes which are excluded from analysis.

For the purpose of this study, two main developments are critical to understand the patterns of policy making under the HTP reform umbrella (a) the introduction of universal health insurance and (b) the digitalization of health services. The main reason for choosing these reforms is that they both have a comprehensive, over sweeping, and innovative nature in the Turkish context. Considering the complexity of issues and the multitude of actors involved in these reforms, policy networks can turn into useful instruments of policy making. However, documentary and field research reveal that neither of these reform processes involved policy networks as defined in this research.

First, the installation of universal health insurance went hand in hand with the general social security reform, two closely intertwined projects launched in 2003. The goal of the general social security reform was to unify three social security institutions (i.e., SSK, Bağ-Kur, and Emekli Sandığı) under the umbrella of one single organization, the Social Security Institution (SSI). In terms of health care, this institutional reconfiguration consisted of a shift from the existing multiple-payer healthcare system managed collectively by the MoH, Ministry of Labor and Social Security, and Ministry of Finance to a single-payer healthcare system managed by the SSI. Universal health insurance coverage was finally achieved on October 1, 2008. The universal health insurance system was installed through close cooperation between three main public institutions including MoH (led by Recep Akdağ as the minister and his design team), SSI (led by Tuncay Teksöz as the founding president of the SSI – a scholar and bureaucrat with extensive experience in healthcare reform), and SPO (known since 2011 as the Ministry of Development). These institutions played a key role in designing universal health insurance, and the two leaders mentioned above can be considered the main policy architects behind the reform.[4]

Prior to universal health insurance reform implementation, a *White Paper on Social Policies*[5] was issued as a product of the:

> co-operation between central economic agencies (the Ministry of Finance, SPO, and the Undersecretariat of Treasury) and spending agencies (the Ministry of Labor and Social Security, the Ministry of Health and the Social Solidarity Fund) for public review and debate. (OECD Economic Surveys: Turkey, 2004, p. 131)

According to the OECD reports, the White Paper on Social Policies "provided a comprehensive account of the fiscal costs of these policies and the results actually obtained. It outlined reform options, with fiscal implications and impacts services" (OECD Economic Surveys: Turkey, 2004). Publication of the White Paper was a ground-breaking policy initiative, witnessed for the first time in Turkish politics.

In the case of Turkey, one motivating force behind issuing a White Paper was the need for data and expertise in the face of the challenging task of revamping the entire social security system. One study has shown that "[t]he Ministry of Health established ongoing collaboration with international agencies and a cadre of national and international experts" and describes the HTP as a "comprehensive strategy informed by evidence" (Atun et al., 2013, p. 71). Yet, in practice, a genuine research community of knowledge-producers with an impact on health policy formulation did not emerge. Hence, instances of policy cooperation and consultation did take the form of expertise-based networks as experienced in the many advanced industrialized countries. In the Turkish case, universal healthcare reforms were the end product of an institutional triad, a form of intra-governmental coordination and planning based on strong team work within and between three public institutions which did not leave much room for non-state

---

[4]See "Universal Health Insurance and the Changing Role of the Ministry of Health" (2007) Ministry of Health, Ankara https://sbu.saglik.gov.tr/Ekutuphane/kitaplar/200801221602180_GSS1.pdf and the article by Alper (2011).

[5]White Papers are critical policy instruments that enable information collection from knowledge-producers including issue area experts, representatives from the academic community, and non-governmental organizations with an interest in the issue. Such information is used to assist policy formulation process. White Papers have been utilized in advanced democracies, particularly in the context of structural reforms with wide socio-economic consequences. For example, the Conservative Party government in the United Kingdom issued a White Paper prior to implementing the 1985 social security reform (Wartonick, 1986, p. 21).

actor intervention. Even though this institutional triad represents an interesting case of inter-governmental level collaboration that deserves further scholarly attention, it does not qualify as a policy networks case as defined in this study.

Secondly, the initiatives of the government to outsource information technology (IT) functions to private companies (i.e., systems integrator firms) within the health sector are referred to as healthcare informatics or digitalization of health care in Turkey. Such initiatives are studied in the context of the digitalization of administrative processes or known as "digital-era governance" (Dunleavy, Margetts, Bastow, & Tinkler, 2006). Constellations of actors working together within this digital platform can be defined as information networks. These networks are composed of governmental and non-governmental actors (i.e., IT companies or non-profit, non-government organizations) that collaborate to build healthcare informatics systems. One concrete example is the collaboration between the MoH, the European Commission, the Software Research and Development Consultancy Limited (SRDC) and healthcare providing institutions in Turkey. The SRDC is founded by a professional team of engineers, located at the Middle East Technical University Technopolis. The aim of establishing this large network is to transfer academic knowledge and know-how as well as build a stronger working relationship among various stakeholders with expertise in the area of e-health. However, these common IT projects can at best be defined as collaborative spaces or collaborative working environments which do not qualify as policy networks with a direct impact on policy making.

Several other IT voluntary associations and private firms have contributed to the digitalization of the healthcare system in Turkey. One of the biggest projects has been the National Health Information System (NHIS) which was launched in 2003 within the framework of the HTP. The NHIS facilitates data (i.e., health records) sharing throughout the country by connecting the MoH to healthcare providers such as hospitals, laboratory systems, and family medicine systems. The NHIS is a nation-wide infrastructure with a centralized architecture that integrates the workings of various actors within the health system (Köse et al., 2008). Due to the very nature of the policy, digitalization of the health system requires the constant communication among many parties with an interest and expertise in the issue. Development of such communication or information networks comes with many opportunities for policy makers and policy practitioners. Studies have shown that demand for new technologies is, in a way, demand for data in policy making, and, subsequently, such information networks can turn into platforms of evidence-based policy making in Turkey (Kahveci & Meads, 2008, p. 238).

However, in spite of instances of consultation, the relation between IT firms and the MoH has been one of outsourcing rather than genuine network collaboration. In this context, large information networks serve as evidence of a systematic centralization or policy reintegration. The digitalization reform in health care is neither an example of network collaboration as defined in this study nor a reversal toward traditional or authoritarian forms of state-controlled governing, often reflected in scholarly circles. Digitalization reforms serve as evidence for re-centralization or re-governmentalization through meta-governance, a specific policy arrangement where the government plays a central role in the coordination of network actors.[6] Such a directed or centralized form of governance becomes particularly important in the management and maintenance of wide-spread networks, including national information systems. As a network increases, it is necessary for one of the actors that has sufficient resources and legitimacy to play a leading role and coordinate relations among all participants (Provan & Kenis, 2008, p. 238; Milward et al., 2009). Otherwise, the network becomes largely ineffective. Hence, digitalization reforms were materialized through collaborative platforms. Yet, such platforms involve operational level collaboration that does not qualify as network policy making where actors are involved into some degree of decision-making with a direct impact on policy making processes.

Both policy reforms have been transformative in terms of achieved outcomes, but not significantly transformative in terms of policy making patterns or the governance side of health. Theoretically, universal healthcare reform illustrates increasing state capacity to deal with challenges confronting public health through intra-governmental coordination mainly between the three institutions (i.e., MoH, SPO, and SSI). Digitalization reforms, on the other hand, represent a case of increasing state capacity though steering IT firms in outsourcing projects. Yet, neither of these reforms consists of devolving responsibility in the sense of including non-state actors into decision-making processes within the health policy area. Both reform processes were initiated and managed by the central government with the MoH as the principal actor in designing and implementing policies. To sum up, the years between 2003 and 2011 can be considered as a period of strong hand governmental intervention through shock therapy reforms. The central government's hands-on approach to health policies was justified on the grounds of missing, and eventually, dire need for reform within the health system in Turkey. Hence, regardless of their centralized nature, implemented health policy reforms were not followed by a wave of substantial criticism or political opposition in the parliament or the mainstream media.

Indeed, HTP reforms represent a continuation in the path of centralized policy making similarly to the pre-2003 period. As stated in the WHO report "the reform process in Turkey has to a large extent been driven by a very strong top-down approach" (WHO, 2012a, p. 25). At the practical level, decision-making was dominated by the MoH and led by a core group of high level bureaucrats and policy experts who worked together as a team (Ağartan, 2005; Atun et al., 2013). Unilateral implementation of the reform package was made possible mainly due to the presence of a strong government with a majority in parliament. Being backed by a "predominant party" (Özbudun, 2014), the government did not lose steam in lengthy and costly consensus building processes like previous coalition governments. Nevertheless, as discussed in the previous section, the central government was experimenting with IT outsourcing and intra-government

[6]The logic provided is similar to the governance experience in the UK during Tony Blair's administration. Reintegration during this period is an example of coordinated governance (i.e., meta-governance) rather than reversal to traditional forms of governing.

coordination which are two different types of governance practices. Due to the presence of such instances of governance, it would be misleading to analyze health policies in Turkey since 2003 as an example of heavy state-controlled policy making or a case for extensive government intervention.

Even though the government engaged in shock therapy reforms that were meant to transform the health system under the HTP reform package, the government still had to prepare the necessary climate for reform legitimation. Certainly, "governance" and "policy collaboration" as generic terms had been incorporated into the jargon of policy making since the early years of HTP program corresponding to the Turkish words "yönetişim" and "sektörler-arası işbirliği," respectively. Legal arrangements made under the provisions of the Public Administration Framework Law can also be read as a governmental attempt to expand the health policy space. This drafted law, vetoed by the President, would have granted financial and administrative authority to the local governments in all policy areas (Tatar et al., 2011). The draft law "would have allowed governance arrangements in the health sector to change significantly, and would have helped to establish quasi-independent units responsible for health sector regulation and public health" (Yasar, 2011). Another drafted law introducing principles for autonomous health enterprises was proposed in 2007 (Yasar, 2011). However, none of these initiatives were enacted into law on the grounds that they would violate the constitution.

Being well aware of the interest groups that would resist the new healthcare initiatives, during the 2003–2010 period, the government effectively managed opposition not through exclusion but through involvement into public debates and platforms which played mostly demonstrative functions with minimal or no impact on policy making (Ağartan, 2005; Sparkes, Bump & Reich, 2015; Duyulmus, 2011). Therefore, networks occupied a place in the rhetoric of public policy. These platforms were far from being inclusive and broad-based with no room for genuine network collaboration though shared decision-making mechanisms. This reality gap has also been reflected in the literature. Some scholars have alluded to the possibility of a "new politics" within the Turkish health policy space but have hesitated to draw any conclusions on a newly emerging collaborative governance (Ağartan, 2005; Wendt, Ağartan, & Kaminska, 2013). According to Wendt, Ağartan and Kaminska, during the implementation of reforms:

> [c]orporate actors have had almost no influence in shaping the reforms because governments … have continued to exclude them from the policy making process and have not incorporated elements of self-regulation into the new governance modes. (2013, p. 94)

As a result, the period between 2003 and 2011 was marked by a duality between (a) the practice of policy making driven by shock therapy response and driven by a "majority government … able to command the support of the legislature" (Tatar & Kavanos, 2006, p. 22) and (b) the emerging policy rhetoric oriented toward new forms of governance. Stated differently, the central government's hands-on approach to health reform management did not prevent the emergence of network thinking within the Turkish public administration. This dual dynamics is reflected in interviews with ministerial and professional experts conducted during field research who repeatedly pointed out a general awareness and rising rhetoric on cross-sectoral collaboration and governance since the introduction of HTP reforms, and yet, missed clear coordinates on how such collaboration would work in practice. Without falling into the trap of linear logic analysis that leads us either toward state-controlled health policy making, on the one hand, or marketization of the health system due to a neo-liberal shift in government policies, on the other hand, it is possible to argue that the post-2003 health system reconfiguration represented new opportunities (1) for re-considering the role, function, and responsibilities of the existing actors including the central government; (2) for the proliferation of new actors with a stake in policy making, especially non-state actors in relatively new policy areas such as health digitalization, biomedical technology, medical industry, public health development, health tourism, community-based health services, etc., and as a natural consequence new opportunities; and (3) for the re-definition of the relations and interactions between actors in the health sector.

Considering the dual dynamics in policy making since 2003, the argument put forward here is that the terms cross-sectoral collaboration (sektörler-arası işbirliği/çok paydaşlı işbirliği modelleri) and governance (yönetişim) entered the policy jargon before they were practically utilized as policy instruments. The new HTP reform package utilized the new policy rhetoric on governance and collaboration even though this program itself was centrally orchestrated and managed. More importantly, the majority of the policy goals under the HTP reform package presumed some degree of responsibility sharing in healthcare services as well as proliferation of actors capable of engaging in different forms of cross-sectoral interactions such as multi-agent negotiations and multi-layered agreements. However, critical questions still remain. Is the policy rhetoric on networks matched by reality? Are actors practically involved in network policy making as defined in this study? Field research shows that policy networks have been involved in health policy making in the critical juncture between 2011 and 2015. The following section aims at understanding the timing as well as factors that led to their emergence in 2011 as well as their demise in 2015. A more detailed account of the nature and structure of policy networks will be discussed in Chapter 4.

Networks as Concrete Policy Instruments (2011–2015)

Despite the growing significance of governance and cross-sectoral collaboration, networks as tools of policy making were not utilized until 2011 which can be considered as a pivotal year for network formation. The year 2011 corresponds to the finalization of the first wave of HTP reforms. The timing of network collaboration within the Turkish heath sector during this time is not a coincidence. This section investigates the motives behind the formation of policy networks by outlining some of the main contextual factors triggering network collaboration, namely (a) multi-faceted health programs, (b) institutional reorganization, and (c) conducive political and social environment.

Policy networks were utilized in the framework of multi-faceted health programs, which were introduced and implemented in Turkey especially after 2011. These programs constituted new directions in health policy, a shift from health policy reforms through major system-level transformations (2003–2010) to health policy development which required policy innovation, policy expertise, and multi-stakeholder coordination (post-2011). Since the initiation of reforms in 2003, the government had anticipated a period of cross-sectoral policy collaboration ensuing the first wave of reforms within the health system. The post-2011 period can be described as a phase of policy reorientation toward new targets in the area of health care. In official government documents, the first wave of reforms is described as a period designed to repair the health system through drastic policy change, whereas the second wave of reforms is described as a period designed to foster policy goals through programs based upon cross-sectoral collaboration (Ministry of Health, 2014, p. 21).

During the first wave of reforms, MoH was chiefly responsible for handling a crisis situation in health care as well as dealing with controversial policy issues such as universal healthcare coverage in a decisive, autonomous, and centralized fashion. The second part of the HTP (post-2011 period) represents a shift toward broad-based actor engagement concerning long-term and multi-faceted policy challenges in relatively new policy sub-areas with the goal of improving public health. Such a shift required information and expertise exchange among multiple stakeholders and above all a new policy kit based on the logic of shared governance though international and inter-sectoral collaboration as well as increased capacity for stewardship (see MoH First Strategic Plan 2010–2014). Moreover, reconfiguration of the health system led to new healthcare needs and challenges of a complex and multi-faceted nature.

Relatively new policy sub-areas within the healthcare system involved extensive multi-actor interactions and potential for collaboration among them. For the purpose of this book I call these policy sub-areas *network domains* (i.e., policy sub-areas that serve as fertile ground for network collaboration). Four network domains can be identified as the following: (1) public health development; (2) medical industry; (3) health tourism; and (4) community-based health and social services. Each policy sub-area involves different actor constellations, and all network prone domains represent promising areas for the study of policy networks due to the large number of involved actors and multi-faceted nature of issues at stake. Hence, network domains serve as fertile ground to explore the emergence of policy networks as policy instruments with some comparative advantages over cumbersome bureaucracies and rivalry-driven markets. These four sub-areas are marked by at least three common attributes:

Multidisciplinary nature of issues: The four network domains cut across policy areas, levels of governance, sectors, and organizations. For instance, health tourism is at the intersection of two main policies, namely health and tourism, and also has an impact on other policy areas such as culture, economic development, education, labor, and social security. Moreover, multiple organizations from the public, private, and voluntary sectors are concerned with the issue of health tourism at the national, regional, and local levels of governance. Another example is public health policy development, the definition of which has shifted from absence of disease (curative health) to general wellbeing (preventive health). The former is covered by hospital services, whereas the latter is much more comprehensive including issues such as clean water, transportation, housing, and community services that cannot be managed by a single governmental body. Gradually, public health has turned into a multi-faceted policy issue that involves multiple stakeholders from different policy sectors and organizations.

Inherent complexity of issues: Another attribute of the four network domains considered in this study is issue complexity. Existing institutions are not equipped to deal separately with high levels of complexity or high levels of risk. Therefore, multiple actors are involved in cross-sectoral collaborative projects. For example, in the area of medical industry, new policies are necessary for the application and management of health technologies in hospitals, bio-technological developments as well as pharmaceutical and medical device innovations. These application spheres require new innovative techniques and assessment methods in addition to the involvement of highly qualified teams including governmental experts, private sector specialists, and professional experts working such as university researchers.

Political salience of issues: At the time of investigation, policy sub-areas under investigation were being kept high on the political agenda which attracted a lot of attention among high level decision-makers at the ministerial level. Some of the policy issues had previously been ungoverned areas, and, therefore, required the establishment of new institutional arrangements such as the public–private partnerships in the healthcare construction sector. Some of the policy issues were considered as projects that promoted Turkey's image abroad (e.g., projects on health tourism). Such projects have a strong political and economic dimension because they serve Turkey's goal of catching up with the advanced industrialized countries and, at the same time, serve as a potential revenue source. Other projects have gained prominence due to the increasing returns on investments in respective policy sub-areas such as medical industry, including biomedical technology programs, and health construction programs. All of these policy sub-areas require collective efforts that cut across narrowly defined policy issues and organizational boundaries, thereby, becoming network prone domains.

The emergence of policy networks was triggered by the expansion of the health system with new policy making actors at the horizontal level. New actors entering the policy space are the end product of an institutional reorganization that was initiated by the executive itself through decree-laws that sped up the administrative reform in health policy management. The year 2011 corresponds to the introduction of KHK No. 663[7] (Resmi Gazete, Vol. 28103, 2011), an executive order that aimed at the reorganization of MoH responsibilities including its role in service provision, finance, and planning as well as expanding the policy space with new regulatory bodies (see Articles 25–30). Particularly important is the formation of subsidiary institutions at the national level including the Turkish Public Health

[7]Statutory Decree No. 663. Published on Official Gazette on November 2, 2011: http://www.resmigazete.gov.tr/eskiler/2011/11/20111102m1-3.htm.

Institute (Türkiye Halk Sağlığı Kurumu), Turkey's Public Hospitals Institution (Kamu *Hastaneleri Birliği Genel Sekreterliği*), and *Turkish Medicines and Medical Devices* Agency (*Türkiye İlaç ve Tıbbi Cihaz Kurumu*). Furthermore, new specialized departments that provide systematic knowledge and expertise in relatively new policy subareas such as Health Investments Directorate (*Sağlık Yatırımları Genel Müdürlüğü*) in the area of public–private partnerships in healthcare construction or General Directorate of Health Development (*Sağlığın Geliştirilmesi Genel Müdürlüğü*) in the area of health tourism were established within MoH. At the local level, besides Provincial Health Directorates (İl *Sağlık Müdürlükleri*), regulatory bodies were established such as Local Public Hospital Institutions (İl Kamu *Hastaneleri Birliği Genel Sekreterliği*) and Local Public Health Directorates (İl Halk Sağlığı Müdürlüğü).

The establishment of these new institutions provides evidence of the shift toward a more dispersed governance of the health policy. Dispersion refers to "fragmentation of policy governance across numerous agencies" (Jenkins & Henry, 2016, p. 709). Unlike decentralization, dispersion does not require a sharp turn in governance patterns or a significant downward power shift. It implies that the decision-making powers are less concentrated in the hands of a few actors within the executive and more dispersed across various governmental offices and agencies. This reorganization of the policy making responsibilities and roles facilitates the formation of collaborative networks within the Turkish health policy space, namely within the policy sub-areas of public health development, health tourism, and healthcare construction.

Devolution of responsibilities at the local level was one of the most groundbreaking administrative reforms carried out within the health system in Turkey, associated with many opportunities, and, at the same time, challenges. Practically, local level devolution consisted of (a) devolving responsibility over implementation of policies at the operational level; (b) devolving partial responsibility over the use of financial resources (over salary budgets through additional payments and the finance of different policy initiatives through approved project proposals); and (c) devolving responsibility over the placement of personnel hired on individual contracts by the institution at the local level (KHK No. 663). This type of institutional devolution or shifting competence toward the local level was certainly conducive to governance of health institutions, facilities, and services, with the potential to serve as ground for network collaboration at the local level. However, the new system was harshly criticized for the lack of clearly defined boundaries about the roles and responsibilities of each organization, and, eventually lack of a clear framework that would regulate interactions among multiple organizations at the local level.[8]

Institutional reorganization and multi-faceted health programs took place within a favorable political and social environment. The argument put forward here is that the 2011–2015 interval is a time period marked by policy legitimacy and also policy stability, where both contribute to an environment conducive to network collaboration, with minimal levels of social tension and political opposition.

[8]The Convention on Healthcare Management. "3. Sağlık Yönetimi Kongresi" Nisan 2015/Ankara https://www.medikalakademi.com.tr/kongre/3-saglik-yonetimi-kongresi/

Legitimacy, here, refers to (a) absence of stark opposition or substantive opposition from political parties, stakeholders, media, and scholarly circles as well as (b) general public satisfaction with the results of the health reforms. Concerning the first, even though there was some opposition, particularly from professional associations which were excluded from the decision-making processes (Ağartan, 2015, 2016), health policy ceased to be a fiercely fought political battle at least for some time. There was an awareness that the first wave of reforms largely met the policy expectations and produced beneficial outcomes for the citizens which created a general atmosphere of reform zeal. Scholarly assessments of reforms have generally been positive putting forward the argument that reforms have achieved considerable levels of success and there is still room for improvement. HTP reform assessments have varied from highly positive accounts focusing on the progress side and specific achievements of the reforms (Akdağ, 2015; Akıncı, Mollahaliloğlu, Gürsöz, & Öğücü, 2012; Atun et al., 2013; Bariş, Mollahaliloğlu, & Aydin, 2011; Chakraborty, 2009; Horton & Lo, 2013; Vujicic, Sparkes, & Mollahaliloğlu, 2009) to many neutral-constructive accounts describing reforms as not having serious technical flaws in their design, recognizing achievements, and highlighting limitations mostly related to reform sustainability in the long run (Ağartan, 2012; Akbulut, Sarp, & Uğurluoğlu, 2007; Aran, & Rokx, 2014; Erus & Aktakke, 2012; Gürsoy, 2015; Ökem & Çakar, 2015; Sahın, Özcan, & Özgen, 2011; Sülkü, 2011; Tatar et al., 2011; Yardim, Çilingiroğlu, & Yardim, 2013; Yıldırım & Yıldırım, 2011). Only a few substantially critical accounts focused on deeply rooted problems of the reforms that immersed the health system into even a deeper crisis than the pre-reform period (Balta, 2013; Belek, 2012; Elveren, 2008; Kilic, 2014; TMA, 2011; Yilmaz, 2013). In addition, international organizations considered the Turkish experience as an example of good practice and remarkable progress (OECD, 2008; WB, 2010; WHO, 2012), a position that contributed toward health reform legitimization.

In spite of criticism from a group of scholars, professional associations, unions, and the main opposition parties, at the end of the first wave of reforms, there was no image of incapacitated government or unproductive reforms among the citizens. On the contrary, reforms were followed by a general public satisfaction (see Fig. 1) which hit record highs in 2010. General public satisfaction was the result of (a) a growing patient satisfaction with the current healthcare facility services offered particularly in population and family health centers followed by public hospitals and university hospitals (Health Statistics Yearbook, MoH, 2010, p. 121); (b) the presence of a relatively young population with lower expectations of health policies (Hazama, 2015); and, finally (c) a prevailing public opinion on successful reform made possible by several framing strategies deployed by the government (Ağartan, 2016). The outcomes of the 2011 elections served as a barometer of the general public support for the reforms implemented thus far. In 2011, the AKP not only won for the third consecutive time but also "won almost twice … the votes of the second-largest party, the CHP (Cumhuriyet Halk Partisi/Republican People's Party) (Özbudun, 2014, p. 156). As recorded by Özbudun (2014), after this landslide victory the AKP became a predominant party that succeeded to consolidate its power. The 2011 elections served a public confidence

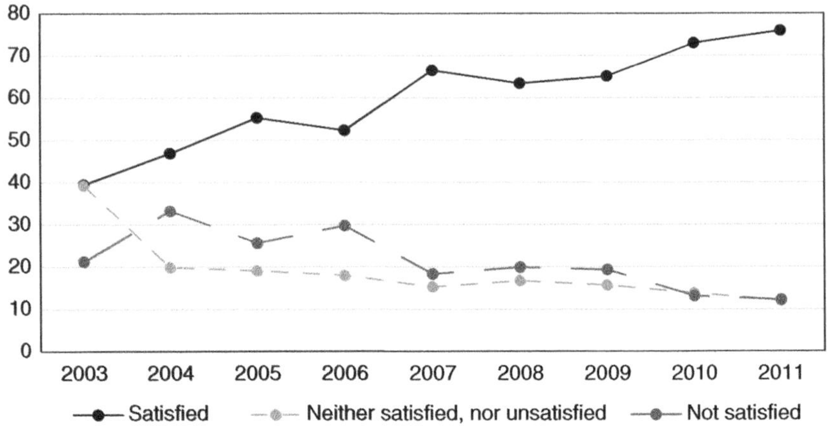

Fig. 1. General Satisfaction with Health Care Services (%), 2003–2010.
Source: TurkStat, Life Satisfaction Survey (2010).

vote that re-enforced the trust in government reform of public services. Amid this consensual atmosphere, the government shifted from building credibility and creating a positive image toward enhancing existing powers by building stronger ties with multiple stakeholders, a situation which naturally paved the way for the formation of policy networks within the health system.

Moreover, the finalization of the reforms in 2011 can be considered as a period of stability referred to as lack of policy change in the literature of comparative public policy. Stability can be understood both in terms of punctuated equilibrium (Baumgartner et al., 2009; Baumgartner & Jones, 2009; Givel, 2010) and in terms of policy stasis (Hirschi & Widmer, 2010; Hope & Raudla, 2012). These are two situations that lead to similar policy outcomes, yet involve different mechanisms that hinder change. Stasis can best be defined as the inability to bring change when it is needed, whereas punctuated equilibrium refers to the attempts to keep the status quo by ruling out the possibility of change. Therefore, "punctuated equilibrium includes periods of stability that are quickly changed by major alterations to the policy system" (Givel, 2010, p, 188). Policy stability in post-2011 Turkey fits better within the punctuated equilibrium approach, referring to a period of stability following structural transformation of the health system. After such drastic policy changes which represent a sharp departure from those of the previous health system, the government is less willing to bring any major policy changes in an attempt to keep the status quo. Reluctance to introduce major policy change could be due to reform fatigue or simply resource depletion.

Nevertheless, in the case of Turkey, the central government reluctance to introduce further policy change of a transformative nature is mainly due to lack of endogenous and exogenous shocks that bring immediate challenges to the existing health system. For example, no immediate policy concerns pointing out detrimental effects of certain health policies or implemented reforms were brought on the table. Similarly, no external pressure or disturbances such as the case of massive refugee inflows that put a significant extra burden on the health system were witnessed until 2015. In this context, the government was more inclined toward creating strategic stakeholder alliances mainly with industry associations and professional associations, which would sustain the status quo by ruling out the possibility of major policy change. Under such circumstances, policy networks serve as instruments that keep the health system intact rather than opportunities to overhaul the health system.

Overall, both policy legitimacy and stability represent contextual conditions that bring state and non-state actors closer in collaborative projects and eventually trigger network formation. Even though scholars tend to focus on causes and consequences of policy change which is at the heart of comparative public policy, this study shows that policy stability is useful to understand the formation stage of policy networks. The Turkish case clearly shows that policy networks do not emerge during times of policy change or transformation that result in major alterations but rather during times of policy stability coupled with considerable amounts of policy legitimacy, where the executive branch of the government is more open toward the idea of devolving responsibilities and duties.

Networks as Unfinished Projects (Post-2015 Period)

The period of stability and legitimacy described above lasted from 2011 to 2015. The second half of 2015 marks the starting point of slowdown and even reversal of cross-sectoral collaboration mainly due to the growing security concerns in Turkish politics as well as growing sustainability concerns within the health system itself. Rising political and social opposition, escalating foreign policy tension, and a general election in 2015 were among the few contextual factors that led the ruling AK Party face a setback and re-think the policy agenda. Acute migration flows crossing the Turkish border constituted a new burden for the health system both in terms of finances and human resources (Döner, Özkara, & Kahveci, 2013). Following the massive refugee influx to Turkey, there were growing concerns about "increasing communicable disease risks, overcrowding hospitals, and more generally straining financial and health resources" (Ekmekci, 2017, p. 1434). According to the Turkish Statistical Institute (TÜİK) the number of patient hospital visits per physician has been recorded as an increasing trend since 2015[9] contributing to growing pressures from within the health system. Growing awareness of the continuing problems within the health policy area as well as rising security concerns external to the health system, such as the spreading securitization discourse and the Syrian refugee crisis, led to the creation of a new political climate which was no longer conducive to relatively costly and lengthy cross-sectoral policy programs.

Since 2015, the political atmosphere in Turkey has been dominated by a growing securitization discourse which was further amplified by the failed coup attempt

[9]Turkish Statistical Institute, Health and Social Protection Dataset: http://tuik.gov.tr/UstMenu.do?metod=temelist.

in July 15, 2016. After this date, the government moved away from the realm of normal politics and entered the realm of extraordinary politics. The failed coup attempt was the turning point toward emergency and power politics that shaped media channels, public opinion, and, most importantly, the public policy agenda. Since then, policy developments have been under the influence of executive orders. For the purpose of this study, publication of KHK 694,[10] is critically important leading to the re-configuration of the health system. This statutory decree resulted in the concentration of power back to MoH which left no room for devolution of responsibility across various institutions at the national and local levels. KHK 694 introduced in 2017 annulled the provisions of KHK 663 based on the grounds of an inefficient system of governance. This governmental provision formally took the Turkish health system to the pre-2011 period due to measures of re-centralization within the health system in line with the redefinition of the role and responsibilities of the MoH. Additionally, MoH took back some of the tasks and responsibilities that had devolved to subsidiary institutions by incorporating them as directorates under the ministry's organizational schema. For instance, Public Health Institute was re-positioned directly under the control of the MoH and re-named as Public Health General Directorate. Against this background, an upward transfer of responsibilities took place causing the disruption of multi-stakeholder policy programs in the area of public health development.

For the purpose of this book, the year 2017 marks the disruption of cross-sectoral collaboration due to (a) policy reversals, (b) institutional re-centralization, and (c) a wide-spread security rhetoric that put an end to the previous atmosphere of trust in the health policy environment. Network collaboration through multi-stakeholder policy platforms and programs flourished in the period between 2011 and 2015 and has slowed down ever since. The presence of these two statutory decrees once more confirms the argument that policy networks are deliberate governmental choices that are initiated as well as terminated under specific political and policy circumstances. Statutory decrees issues in 2011 and 2017 hold symbolic value, the significance of which stands in marking the begging and the end of a golden age of network collaboration during which the central government engaged in broad actor coalitions and alliances with the purpose of maintaining the post-reform status quo within the health policy area.

To sum up, the second wave of reforms under the HTP corresponded to temporary adaptation in policy making patterns through the formation of policy networks in the five-year period lasting from 2011 to 2015. Newly emerging network collaboration was based on the logic of dispersing responsibilities to other stakeholders within the healthcare system through various cross-sectoral arrangements at different stages of policy making. These cross-sectoral projects were managed by new regulatory agencies and governmental bodies specialized in new areas of policy making within the health system. Despite their significance, the networks

[10]Statutory Decree No. 694 was issued under the State of Emergency (OHAL) on August 15, 2017 and published in the Official Gazette on August 25, 2017: http://www.resmigazete.gov.tr/eskiler/2017/08/20170825-13.pdf.

under investigation constitute venues of temporary policy experimentation rather than instruments of genuine institutional transformation. Field research shows that systematic structures and legal frameworks that would facilitate the institutionalization of network collaboration as a pattern of governance in the long run are largely missing. The interruption of network collaboration after 2015, particularly within the fields of health tourism and public health, shows that policy networks could not become firmly established policy instruments. Policy networks that fell short of reaching the stage of institutional consolidation were utilized to achieve short-term objectives within the framework of cross-sectoral collaboration.

Conclusion

There is too much focus on the design and structure of policy networks (i.e., spatial dimension) rather than the pathways of network formation or how policy networks come into being (i.e., time dimension). This chapter contributes to the debates on network formation by exploring the conditions under which networks form within the Turkish health system through a retrospective health policy analysis. This chapter presents an account of network formation by focusing on when and why policy networks emerge in a policy setting with a tradition of centralized and hierarchical decision-making. Two essentially interlinked questions are addressed here in an attempt to understand the context of network formation.

Concerning the "when" question, this chapter shows that policy networks do not emerge during times of sharp policy change which are orchestrated single-handedly by specialized and focused teams within the central government, more specifically the MoH in Turkey. Both desk and field research reveal that during the first years of the HTP reform processes, terms such as cross-sectoral collaboration and governance entered the policy making jargon and became quite popular. However, they did not materialize in concrete policy instruments and practices. In the period from 2011 to 2015, new institutional arrangements were established by the government itself to steer and manage the interaction with other non-governmental actors in policy sub-areas, such as public health development, medical industry, and health tourism. For the purpose of this chapter, the 2011–2015 period can be considered as a critical juncture for the temporary emergence of network collaboration within the health policy area.

Hence, policy networks emerged during times of policy stability and legitimacy including both crucial conditions for maintenance of an atmosphere of trust among stakeholders. Under such circumstances governmental actors are more willing to cooperate and share governance responsibilities with public, private, and voluntary actors. Stability and legitimacy should not be perceived as necessary conditions but rather as background conditions that explain collaboration within the Turkish health policy space. This study suggests that the analysis of policy networks should be contextualized (i.e., one should closely examine causal mechanisms and the context in which policy networks operate – an important step for building middle-range theories in comparative public policy studies, and more specifically for contributing to debates on network formation) (see Falleti & Lynch, 2009, for the role of context and contextual mechanisms).

Concerning the "why" question, this study shows that policy networks are first and foremost governmental choices made under certain political and economic crosscurrents. Hence, the presence of policy networks in the case of Turkey indicates that networks are not an inevitable course of action, as often presented in the context of advanced democracies, but an institutional arrangement often generated and managed by the government itself. Policy networks are not natural occurrences, they are deliberate governmental choices utilized, maintained, or even dissolved due to changing political and policy priorities.

The analysis further reveals that contextual factors bolster government choice to engage in cross-sectoral collaboration. This chapter suggests that policy networks are formed primarily due to the combination of three contextual factors which reinforce each other and contribute to network formation. These are (a) policy shift toward multi-faceted policy programs, (b) institutional reorganization that bring about devolution of responsibilities across a larger number of actors within the health system, and finally (c) a conducive political and social environment marked by policy stability and legitimacy. In the cases under consideration, policy networks emerge in times of policy stability and legitimacy, when the government tended to maintain the current status quo through partnerships and relatively broad and inclusive collaborative projects.

At a more theoretical level, this chapter suggests that policy networks are neither public policy panaceas designed to deal with wicked or complex problems as functionalists would argue nor natural and inevitable consequences of private and voluntary actor empowerment, as the network governance perspective would suggest, at least not in the strictest sense. Subsequently, the view that policy networks are institutional structures that emerge naturally and evolve gradually in the form of linear progression toward governance is simply untenable. When it comes to the rationale of their formation, policy networks are contingent and optional rather than inevitable and necessary in nature. Hence, networks can best be conceived as policy instruments deliberately utilized by the government under specific political, institutional, and policy conditions.

Finally, it is worth noting that the formation of policy networks does not guarantee their continuity. Against this background, it is important to examine the internal structure as well as institutional resilience of policy networks. The following chapter will focus on 2011–2015 period which can be considered a pivotal juncture for network policy making in Turkey in an attempt to understand the dynamics of collaboration within policy networks under investigation. Further questions should be considered in the study of these policy networks include the following: What is the structure of interaction within policy networks? Do scholars observe genuine network collaboration as symmetrical (i.e., structure of collaboration), integrated (i.e., trust based), and durable (i.e., institutionalized) systems of cooperation among network participants similar to advanced industrialized countries? Alternatively, do scholars observe self-interested actors constantly competing for funding and other resources in the form of occasional, shallow, loose, and fragmented cooperation without a common vision and shared goals? These questions as well as others will be addressed in the following chapters.

Chapter 4

Becoming Collaborative: Policy Networks within the Turkish Health Sector in Turkey

Abstract

This chapter examines factors that maximize collaboration among various stakeholders with the purpose of health policy making in Turkey. The field research reveals that policy networks have been formed in the sub-areas of public health, healthcare construction, and health tourism in the years between 2011 and 2015. Content analysis of 24 semi-structured interviews with policy and professional experts is conducted to assess Network Collaborative Capacity, built upon three dimensions, namely, structural, relational, and institutional. The findings reveal that networks differ in their capacity to collaborate as well as their impact on policy making resulting in three distinct models of network policy making. In the cases under investigation, network impact takes the form of (a) policy innovation through expertise sharing and evidence-based policy making associated with particularly high levels of relational capacity; (b) policy effectiveness through contract enforcement within a clear legal framework associated with particularly high levels of institutional capacity; and (c) policy coherence through organizational-knowledge-sharing and actor coordination. Findings also suggest that institutionalization in the form of network embeddedness in the surrounding political and economic environment is crucial for maintaining a collaborative momentum as well as achieving policy effectiveness at the stage of policy implementation. Based on these findings, further studies should focus on the institutionalization of policy networks, particularly in those middle-income countries such as Turkey that aim and often fail to address various policy challenges through short-lived practices of multi-stakeholder action. Finally, this study emphasizes the importance of incorporating neo-institutional approaches to network analysis.

Keywords: Network collaborative capacity (NCC); content analysis; health sector; network embeddedness; policy networks; Turkey

---

Network Policy Making within the Turkish Health Sector. Becoming Collaborative, 63–93

doi:10.1108/978-1-83867-094-820201005

> [...] the quality of collaborations has rarely been investigated in a structured or systematic way. (Bennett, Glandon, & Rasanathan, 2018, p. 1)

In one of his seminal works, Robert Agranoff (2006) points out that "[t]he network is not the only vehicle of collaborative management" (p. 57). There is a plethora of "collaborative endeavors" (Agranoff, 2006, p. 57). This study focuses exclusively on policy networks which are not perceived superior forms of collaboration but are viewed as vehicles of collaboration with a more direct or measurable policy impact that can be investigated empirically. Other forms of stakeholder involvement without direct influence on policy making (e.g., dialogue committees, advisory councils, informal meetings with heads of government, public campaigns, and advocacy or discourse coalitions) can barely be measured empirically. One important feature that distinguishes policy networks from other forms of collaborative endeavors is "the production of a common outcome" (Börzel, 1998, p. 264) which allows this form of policy collaboration to be investigated empirically in a more structured and systematic way through a close examination of policy making processes. Against this background, the aim of this chapter is to focus on network practices present within the Turkish health sector and assess their capacity to facilitate collaboration among multiple stakeholders with some impact on policy making processes.

Field research conducted in Turkey in the year 2015 reveals that collaborative endeavors within the health sector are numerous. Even though their practical significance is now being acknowledged, at the theoretical level, all instances of inclusive policy making that involve non-state actors are lumped together under the generic term cross-sectoral collaboration translated to Turkish as "sektörler arası işbirliği" or "çok paydaşlı işbirliği çalışmaları."[1] Therefore, the real challenge has been to distinguish policy networks from other cross-sectoral arrangements that have failed to become collaborative. The first task of this research has been to provide a clear, concise, and value-free definition that would reflect the complexity of network collaboration as a concept while simultaneously guiding field research through a set of concrete, measurable, and standardized criteria that distinguish network type of collaboration in practice. Based on the definition provided in this study, three operationalizable criteria have been used to identify and distinguish policy networks: first, policy networks must be cross-sectoral, meaning that they must involve stakeholders from public, private, and voluntary sectors (i.e., network input). Second, policy networks must facilitate recurring interaction within the policy making cycle, meaning that they involve repetitive and regular activities and tasks spread out over a period of time rather than ad hoc or sporadic encounters (i.e., network processes). Third, policy networks must have some policy impact, meaning that interaction must finalize with some

[1]For more information about the recent debates on cross-sectoral collaboration within the health sector in Turkey, see Özkan (2018). https://www.turkiyeklinikleri.com/upload/issuecontent/halksagligiozel4-2-18.pdf.

collective outcomes that influence or shape policy making processes (i.e., network consequences).

Based on the definition provided above, only a few cross-sectoral encounters within the health sector qualify as policy networks which bring together public, private, and/or voluntary actors distinguished by recurring interactions that influence policy making processes. Policy networks have been formed within three policy sub-areas within the health sector, namely (a) public health (Program for Improving *Multi-Sectoral Health* Responsibility, ÇPSSGP),[2] (b) medical industry (public–private partnerships, PPPs), and (c) health tourism (Health Tourism Coordination Council, SATURK).[3] The goal of this chapter is to scrutinize these policy networks on a case-by-case basis through a detailed assessment of their collaborative capacity, that is, Network Collaborative Capacity (NCC), a composite index built upon three main measures, namely, structural, relational, and institutional capacity. In the three policy sub-areas under consideration, 28 semi-structured interviews (24 interviews have been audio-recorded) have been conducted with policy and professional experts representing central and local government organizations, semi-public organizations, industry associations, professional associations, service oriented community organizations, and universities active within the field of health. A detailed account of the sample of organizations, interview questions, and coding used in content analysis are provided in the Appendix. The results of the content analysis are summarized in Table 4 and discussed in the following sections.

Program for Improving *Multi-Sectoral Health* Responsibility (ÇPSSGP)

Network Policy Background

The global trends in the area of public health have been in favor of preventive health or general wellbeing that keeps the citizens away from overloaded hospital services and ensures healthier lifestyles particularly in the urban settings. International and regional organizations such as World Health Organization (WHO) and the European Union (EU) have provided policy directives and guidelines as well as funds supporting collaborative projects that promote the involvement of municipalities, non-governmental organizations (NGOs), and other local actors with a stake in the development of public health policies. The establishment of the "European Healthy Cities Network" initiated approximately 30 years ago best illustrates this approach to public health.

> Health in all policies is based on a recognition that population health is not merely a product of health sector activities but largely determined by policies and actions beyond the health sector.

[2]Çok Paydaşlı Sağlık Sorumluluğunu Geliştirme Programı.
[3]Sağlık Turizmi Koordinasyon Kurulu.

Table 4. Results of Content Analysis.

Network Collaborative Capacity-Categories	**ÇPSSGP**	**PPP**	**SATURK**
1. Inclusiveness	0.60	0.40	0.80
2. Connectedness	0.85	0.37	0.37
2.1 Continuing interaction	0.70	0.50	0.50
2.2 Face-to-face communication	1.00	0.25	0.25
3. Common decision-making	0.60	0.20	0.20
4. Interdependence	0.50	0.87	0.37
4.1 Resource pooling	0.50	0.75	0.25
4.2 Binding rules and regulations	0.50	1.00	0.50
5. Horizontal coordination	1.00	0.05	0.20
5.1 Equal bargaining power	1.00	0.10	0.40
5.2 Efficient self-coordination	1.00	0.00	0.00
STRUCTURAL CAPACITY	0.73*	0.40	0.36
1. Inter-organizational trust	1.00	0.75	0.50
4.1 Willingness to cooperate	0.25	0.25	0.25
4.2 Goal convergence	0.25	0.25	0.25
4.3 Team work	0.25	0.25	0.00
4.4 Synergy	0.25	0.00	0.00
2. Inter-personal trust	1.00	0.00	0.50
RELATIONAL CAPACITY	1.00**	0.37	0.50
1. Media discourse/global/EU policy agenda	0.25	0.25	0.25
2. Prominent political actors/high level officials	0.00	0.25	0.25
3. Existing coalitions/alliances	0.00	0.25	0.00
4. Legislation/formal institution	0.00	0.25	0.12
INSTITUTIONAL CAPACITY	0.25	1.00***	0.62
Average network collaborative capacity	0.66	0.59	0.49

Note:

* This network displays a high score of structural capacity.

** This network displays a high score of relational capacity.

*** This network displays a high score of institutional capacity.

> Health and well-being are increasingly becoming shared values across societal sectors. Solid evidence shows that the actions of other sectors beyond the boundaries of the health sector significantly influence the risk factors of major diseases and the determinants of health. Health in all policies addresses all policies such as those influencing transport, housing and urban development, the environment, education, agriculture, fiscal policies, tax policies and economic policies. (Tsouros, 2009, p. 2)

The implementation of this over-sweeping project initiated by the WHO goes beyond the strict definition of government-led public policy and depends on the collective effort of citizens, politicians, public sector officials, private sector firms, and other agencies interested in addressing public health challenges at the national and local levels. Construction of healthy cities, as envisioned by the WHO, is a globally spread but locally implemented movement of urban lifestyle transformation. The WHO project aims at improving the cities' health profile by reorganizing urban space, redefining citizen lifestyle, revisiting human developmental goals, and introducing a new logic of network governance to public health. Construction of healthy cities is only one example that illustrates how public health policy development goes beyond one single policy domain and requires cross-sectoral collaboration among a multitude of actors at different levels of governance.

Besides the impact of international and regional institutions, the attention of Turkish government on public health issues has increased particularly since 2011. Public health issues did not rank high on the political agenda immediately after the implementation of the HTP in 2003. This was due to the large number of pressing health issues that had to be addressed, such as the reformation of the social security system and the introduction of universal health coverage. However, new healthcare challenges including aging population, growing demand for rehabilitation services, rising healthcare costs, rising rates of chronic disease, insufficient hospital infrastructure, and air and water pollution in the cities were increasingly imposing their toll on the existing healthcare system. Therefore, since 2011, new institutional arrangements have been founded and more financial resources have been directed toward public health-related issues particularly toward projects that follow a holistic and preventive approach to health. The Public Health Institute, with numerous affiliated institutions at the local level, has been the primary agency responsible for improving public health in Turkey in the period 2011–2017. While designing public health policy goals, the government has made use of existing WHO and EU action plans that follow multi-sectoral approaches to policy making.[4] According to the Strategic Plan of the Ministry of Health (MoH) in Turkey, applying a multi-sectoral approach to policy making is necessary to address social

[4]For instance, the *European Action Plan for Strengthening Public Health Capacities and Services* has served as a blueprint for developing the objectives of the *Strategic Plan of the Ministry of Health* in the 2013–2017 period. For more information see https://sgb.saglik.gov.tr/Dkmanlar/Strategic%20Plan%202013-2017.pdf.

determinants of health and reduce health disparities based on the principle of equity (Strategic Plan of the Ministry of Health, 2012, p. 80).

The best case to illustrate multi-sectoral approach to policy making within the area of public health policy development in Turkey is the Program for Improving *Multi-Sectoral Health* Responsibility (Çok Paydaşlı Sağlık Sorumluluğunu Geliştirme Programı/ÇPSSGP). This program constitutes a networked form of collaboration built upon close government–university partnership in the area of public health. Preliminary preparations for the program started in 2009; however, network collaboration, as defined in this study, took place in the years between 2011 and 2013 within the framework of ÇPSSGP. This three-year period served the purpose of designing a comprehensive policy model implementable to various domains of public health. Network collaboration under ÇPSSGP resulted in the development of two main actionable policy plans: (1) The Multisectoral Approach to Health Protection and Promotion (12 policy components and 43 policy sub-components) and (2) The Multisectoral Approach to Curative and Rehabilitative Services (8 policy components and 16 policy sub-components). The overarching goals of this comprehensive program are to identify and tackle some of the most recent challenges to public health particularly in the urban settings and build national as well as local level capacity to implement policy objectives in the area of public health by adopting a multi-sectoral approach.

Network Structure

As stated in previous chapters, network structural capacity is measured against five components: (a) inclusiveness, (b) connectedness, (c) common decision-making, (d) interdependence, and (e) horizontal coordination which serve as categories in the content analysis of the interview transcripts. ÇPSSGP records a relatively high score of structural capacity (0.73/1.00) compared to other network cases under investigation.

In terms of inclusiveness, ÇPSSGP represents a broad network composed of representatives from more than 100 institutions and agencies. ÇPSSGP included representatives from 33 universities dispersed geographically throughout Turkey. As noted in the project's final report, the program was based upon the close collaboration of 759 representatives including 235 scholars, 138 experts from the MoH, and 386 public health professionals and experts from other institutions.[5] Even though ÇPSSGP is a very broad network in terms of actor composition, the close cooperation between three partner institutions and their corresponding teams is at the heart of this network and key to understanding the peculiar dynamics of the network under consideration. These are the team led by the MoH[6] primarily responsible for actor coordination (i.e., planning and supervision, logistics

[5]More information on the names of the organizations that participated in the program can be found under the following link https://hsgm.saglik.gov.tr/depo/birimler/cevre-sagligi/1-su-guvenligi/Kitaplar/CokPaydaslisaglsorgelisProOzet_Kitap.pdf.

[6]Public Health Institute, Environmental Health Department, affiliated with the MoH played a very important role in the management of the ÇPSSGP.

operation, activity management, and intra-network communication), the team led by the Ministry of Development primarily responsible for financial coordination (i.e., resource management), and the team led by the Düzce University primarily responsible for program coordination (i.e., scientific/technical coordination).

The Düzce University team which represents the intellectual backbone of the program in collaboration with researchers from other universities in Turkey is particularly important for the purpose of this study. University researchers can be perceived as academic or civil society entrepreneurs who played a crucial role in the initiation of the program in the first place, existing in close cooperation with government experts working in the Institute of Public Health in Turkey. Other civil society representatives such as NGOs are of secondary importance and almost non-existent at the decision-making stage of the ÇPSSGP. In the case of ÇPSSGP, NGOs regain importance as critical policy making actors only at the implementation stage rather than early stages of policy making. Overall, ÇPSSGP is the combined effort of three teams mentioned above and their leaders with authoritative roles equally valuable for network management and coordination. This trilateral network structure precludes public authorities from acting as hegemons in the sense of controlling or dominating decision-making processes – a situation that would impair network dynamics.

Particularly important for the purpose of this study are the policy workshops which took the form of expertise exchange labs. According to the interviewees, these workshops were productive venues where participants could spend time together and engage in face-to-face communication which turned out to be very effective in bonding network participants through continuing interaction within relatively small settings. ÇPSSGP policy workshops were designed to work through small, focused, and compartmentalized groups which have some comparative advantages over large fora of dialogue or deliberation. Small specialized groups cover a greater scope of policy issues, avoid thematic overlaps, and facilitate close interaction among their members. Despite being separated into specialized work groups, network participants were not completely detached from each other. Sometimes, one network participant was involved in more than one work group, adding to the overall connectedness of network participants. However, at the end of the day, participants were primarily focused on the policy objectives of their corresponding work groups.

Besides connectedness, small group settings are conducive to common decision-making among their members. As stated in previous research "a small group consists of more than two people who have a perception of common goals, a network communication, some interdependence, some shared norms, and a sense of wholeness" (Gastil, 1993, p. 6). This definition entails that small groups have distributed decision-making power and are essentially democratic in nature. Based on the analysis of the interview transcripts, ÇPSSGP work groups have a similar setting to the definition provided above, and therefore, they score high in terms of common decision-making. The best evidence for the presence of common decision-making is the ability of the work groups to design achievable policy goals. In the end of the collaboration process, participants reach to some sort of common policy understanding and a concrete policy model of public health.

Participants are bonded by some degree of interdependence based upon the exchange of intangible resources. In other words, network participants are bounded by knowledge interdependence in the form of information and expertise sharing rather than sharing of material resources. The structure of interaction within the workshops allowed for the flow of information as well as the effective use of the information in the form of expertise exchange during the policy design stage which was then translated into actionable policy plans. During the workshops group members focus on practical and technical policy related issues instead of engaging in unnecessary and counterproductive political debates. Network participants make use of their professional knowledge and expertise on the issue and do not follow any predetermined policy positions assigned by their organizations. Under such conditions, network participants stop pursuing their own organizational mission over time, acknowledging the benefits of expertise sharing and team work. Thus, ÇPSSGP consists of specialized, task driven, and knowledge intensive work groups which are composed of professionally autonomous actors that depend on each other for achieving common policy goals.

Overall, the degree of interdependence between participating actors is on average levels. In other words, network members are able to maintain strong reciprocal relations nourished by mutual exchange of mainly intangible resources (i.e., information and expertise exchange), agree on the terms and conditions of the collaborative project from the start (i.e., *ex ante* organizational rules), and have a mutual understanding of rules of operation but lack any form of economic interdependence (i.e., observed in co-finance or co-investment project/programs) and *ex post* rules of enforcement concerning the outcomes of the decision-making process.

Finally, ÇPSSGP scores high in terms of horizontal coordination among participants. Work groups facilitate the mutual exchange of ideas among their participants regardless of their position, status, and organizational affiliation. In the case of ÇPSSGP, network participants are constantly exchanging information and they are capable of negotiating with each other on an equal level contributing to relatively high levels of horizontal coordination (i.e., equal bargaining power). In addition, network participants are involved in decentered interaction which is made possible by the network structure itself. The presence of a trilateral network structure makes it possible for all the three teams to equally contribute toward policy development through mechanisms of horizontal coordination within a relatively flat network structure. Last but not least, the presence of a computer modeling as a policy tool useful for recording and tracking workshop outcomes contributed to efficient self-coordination of the network.

Overall, ÇPSSGP scores high levels of structural capacity contributing to high levels of expertise and knowledge-sharing, and, eventually policy innovation. This network is a highly integrated web of actors with similar educational and professional backgrounds. Structurally, the network operating under ÇPSSGP can be considered as a *compartmentalized policy network* with small work groups operating within the program. This type of setting facilitates horizontal coordination among actors contributing to high levels of collaboration.

Intra-network Relations

ÇPSSGP exhibits a particularly high score of relational capacity or the capacity to facilitate trust-based interaction among participants. Trust-based interaction is a function of actors' (a) willingness to cooperate, (b) goal convergence, (c) team work, and (d) synergy. Content analysis reveals that these components were all present in the ÇPSSGP work groups amounting to a maximum score in terms inter-organizational trust. Words such as "shared vision" and "team spirit" were frequently reiterated by the interviewees as the engine behind collaboration in the ÇPSSGP program. Naturally, a shared vision is necessary to kindle enthusiasm and solidarity among participants and to motivate them to work together. Team environment, on the other hand, is necessary to foster synergy among network participants and eventually lead to brainstorming and policy innovation. Interviewees reveal that team environment was not present from the onset of collaboration, instead it was developed gradually due to the work and constant efforts of project coordinators who played a critical role in building an environment of trust around network participants.

ÇPSSGP work groups played a critical role in developing trust, bridging organizational divides, and building a team environment and maintaining group solidarity. Hence, ÇPSSGP work groups turned into ideal settings for synergetic team work among professionals representing different organizations and eventually lead to the development of inter-organizational trust. Interviewees agree that in the case of ÇPSSGP, network interaction started with a trust vacuum that gradually developed during the collaborative process. It is also worth mentioning that the presence of inter-organizational trust does not guarantee the total absence of friction or confrontation between organizations. Yet, the bottom line here is that confrontation does not turn into irresolvable conflict. The case of ÇPSSGP demonstrates that small group interaction minimizes the incompatibilities or conflicts that emerge occasionally. Additionally, clear organizational rules agreed at the beginning of collaboration are helpful to keep conflict at bay.

Notably, work groups operating under ÇPSSGP enabled close, frequent, and face-to-face communication among participants which contributed to the evolution of semi-informal relations. Interviewees agreed that face-to-face communication within these small work groups was important in increasing the effectiveness of the decision-making process and engendering network cohesiveness. Here, a close relationship does not entail the presence of informal relations among network participants which can even be detrimental to network effectiveness and professional interaction. The interviewees reveal that network participants were bonded by a close and professional relationship with each other which continued even after the project was completed. Hence, it is possible to conclude that network interaction within the ÇPSSGP work teams was *carried* out in a semi-formal fashion that led to the development of interpersonal trust among network participants with a similar professional background.

Network Institutionalization

Network institutionalization is defined as network embeddedness in the surrounding political, economic, and policy environment or anchorage of the network in the external environment. Network embeddedness or institutionalization contributes to overall collaborative capacity by sheltering the network from external influences that could adversely affect network dynamics and entrenching the network in the existing policy environment. Four measures have been used to gauge network institutionalization in this study: (a) presence of prevailing policy discourse; (b) support from prominent political actors or high level bureaucrats in the government; (c) existing coalitions or interest-based alliances; and (d) presence of government departments or other formal institutions concerning the policy issue at hand. As it is demonstrated in Table 4 ÇPSSGP exhibits a low score of institutionalization (0.25/1.00).

ÇPSSGP represents a case of policy collaboration where participants have been more preoccupied with maintaining intra-network, trust-based relations and less preoccupied with building extra-network, strategic linkages that would facilitate network sustainability in the long run. The program follows the WHO and EU public health policy targets, and therefore, serves as a legitimate platform for public health policy development. Nevertheless, there is a common understanding among interviewees that the political support and governmental willingness to implement policy proposals were largely lacking. Even though ÇPSSGP complies with global and regional policy discourse, it did not rank high in the domestic policy and political agenda. Previous research has shown that "political priority is considered a facilitating factor to the success of addressing public health issues" (Hoe, Rodriguez, Üzümcüoğlu, & Hyder, 2016). For example, the success of the National Tobacco Control Program[7] in the area of public health is often explained by the fact that this program turned into the political priority of the Turkish government in the period between 2008 and 2012 (Hoe et al., 2016; Hoe, Rodriguez, Üzümcüoğlu, & Hyder, 2019).

ÇPSSGP resulted in the production of 12 action plans, which constitute a good opportunity for the promotion of public health in Turkey. However, the suggested policy model, based on the idea of cross-sectoral collaboration at the community level, did not receive the necessary political and financial support from the upper levels of decision-making in the executive branch of the government needed to push the model forward to the implementation stage. The lack of external anchorage in the political and economic environment clearly explains the

[7]The National Tobacco Control Program was carried out in the years between 2008 and 2012. MoH and the Tobacco and Alcohol Market Regulatory Authority (TAP-DK) with the assistance of the WHO are the main institutions responsible for the implementation and monitoring of the program. These institutions were supported by other governmental departments and agencies including Ministry of Industry and Trade, Ministry of Finance, the Radio and Television Supreme Council, Ministry of the Interior, State Airports Administration, Ministry of Finance, and Ministry of Agriculture and Rural Affairs. Even though the program received strong support by NGOs and academics, it remains a government initiative based on inter-agency collaboration, and, therefore, it is not treated as a case of network collaboration in this study. For more information on the program, see Bilir, Çakır, Dağlı, Ergüder, and Önder (2009).

relatively short life of the network collaboration under ÇPSSGP which, regardless of its unprecedented success at the stage of policy design and formulation, failed to produce practical outcomes with tangible impact on the health of citizens in Turkey. The ÇPSSGP case once more proves the argument of network reliance on external support, particularly prior to the policy implementation phase. This phase of policy making requires some extra effort from network participants in order to overcome collaboration fatigue as well as external support needed during the policy implementation stage through funding and/or establishment of additional institutional bodies. Besides the lack of support from the central government, in this case the MoH, the bottom-up advocacy mechanisms that would lead to the adoption of a certain policies are largely lacking adding further to the procrastination of policy implementation.

Three years after the finalization of the policy action plans by the ÇPSSGP, the High Council of Multisectoral Health Responsibility (2017) was formed, composed of Inter-ministerial Executive Boards, the Ministry of Health Coordination Committee, and a Multisectoral Health Responsibility Implementation Coordinator as well as their corresponding sub-committees.[8] The idea behind this Council is to follow a holistic or whole-of-government approach in achieving public health policy goals. The main responsibilities of the Council are to supervise effective policy implementation and facilitate cooperation across various governmental organizations. The Council has been established to contribute to the implementation of the action plans by coordinating inter-ministerial action and bridging different institutional needs. On paper, the Council serves as an instrument that catalyzes policy implementation though close inter-agency coordination within the government. When established in 2017, the Council consisted of the Prime Minister's Office as a lead actor together with Minister of Family and Social Policies, Minister of Science, Industry and Technology, Minister of Labor and Social Security, Minister of Environment and Urban Planning, Minister of Foreign Affairs, Minister of Youth and Sports, Minister of Internal Affairs, Minister of Development, Minister of Culture and Tourism, Minister of Development, Minister of National Education, and Minister of Health.

Despite its significance as an inter-agency coordination Council, there are doubts about its effectiveness in practice. The Council under investigation meets annually which makes it difficult to overcome collective action problems and coordinate action across ministerial departments. In terms of policy achievements and outcomes the progress has been too slow. To date, only the Multistakeholder Action Plan on Non-communicable Diseases has been formulated which represents only one among 12 action plans developed by the ÇPSSGP (for more detailed information see MoH, 2017). Consequently, the Council risks deviating

---

[8] MoH, General Directorate of Public Health, Department of Environmental Health: https://hsgm.saglik.gov.tr/tr/cevresagligi-suguvenligi/su-g%C3%BCvenli%C4%9Five-kapl%C4%B1calar-birimi/447-%C3%A7ok-payda%C5%9Fl%C4%B1sa%C4%9Fl%C4%B1k-sorumlulu%C4%9Funu-geli%C5%9Ftirme-program%C4%B1.html. Accessed on June 21, 2019.

from the network logic of policy by emphasizing inter-agency coordination too much within the central government, particularly among ministerial departments, and neglecting adequate levels of interaction with external stakeholders including NGOs and local level actors.

Network Policy Impact

From a governance perspective, ÇPSSGP represents an advanced platform of policy collaboration, where members are bonded to each other by strong ties manifested in the form of synergetic team work (i.e., high levels of relational capacity) within a robust network structure (i.e., high levels of structural capacity). ÇPSSGP best illustrates a type of network collaboration that contributes toward highly innovative policy making in the area of public health at the national level with no other precedent within the health sector in Turkey. ÇPSSGP is a successful model of collaboration which sets a high standard of health policy making. For comparison purposes, a parallel can be drawn between the policy network formed under ÇPSSGP and the ideal type of network interaction elaborated largely by Rod Rhodes (1992, 1997, 2007) in his seminal works. In his studies, Rhodes refers mainly to the British model of collaborative policy making, where highly professional and integrated policy communities, composed of actors with shared interests that work toward common goals. Similarly, ÇPSSGP is composed of governmental experts and academics with similar professional backgrounds in the area of public health who work closely within small group settings that facilitate expertise exchange.

Collaboration under ÇPSSGP takes the form of *health policy hubs* which are common practices of policy making in many developed countries such as Australia, the UK, or the US. Health policy hubs emerge at the early phases of policy making with the purpose of policy design. Technically, health policy hubs contribute to (a) policy innovation and (b) methodological policy development which are intertwined yet separate policy objectives. Policy innovation is expected to take place particularly in the fields of preventive disease, medical devices, and other areas of cutting-edge technology that have a huge impact on public health. The constant pressure toward policy innovation in the area of public health has not only changed the "dynamics of health in a society" but also changed "the mechanisms though which we conduct health policy" as well as "redefine[d]who should be involved in the policy process" (Kickbusch, 2009, p. 1). Methodological development, on the other hand, concerns policy development based upon scientific and statistical data as well as the latest technological advancements within the health sector in Turkey (Kahveci & Meads, 2008). In scientific terminology, methodological policy development is known as evidence-based approach to public health often applied through techniques such as Health Technology Assessment (Lehoux, Denis, Tailliez, & Hivon, 2005).

Network collaboration taking place under the ÇPSSGP has accomplished both policy objectives mentioned above. ÇPSSGP is an example of network collaboration between state bureaucrats and university researchers with expertise in the field of public health policy development in early stages of policy making. This network is nurtured by the strong entrepreneurial impulse of individual actors within the government (i.e., experts working in public offices) and particularly outside the government (i.e., academics), where actors involved aim at bringing change through innovative policy solutions within the area of public health. The role of academics as entrepreneurs contributing toward policy innovation should be highlighted here. Academic entrepreneurs generate pioneering ideas and contribute to the policy design stage through sharing research evidence and professional expertise with governmental authorities. Therefore, interaction takes place mostly at the ideational level and is purely driven by motives of policy innovation rather than gain of tangible benefits. The role of academics can best be defined as "public entrepreneurs who, from outside the formal positions of government, introduce, translate, and help implement new ideas into public practice" (Roberts & King, 1991, p. 147).

In more concrete terms, academic entrepreneurs in the case of ÇPSSGP contribute toward policy innovation primarily through a renewed approach to public health that incorporates prevention and rehabilitation services into the existing healthcare system in Turkey. Policy innovation here is not strictly technological or product based but introduces new standards to public health through knowledge dissemination, awareness rising, and expertise exchange that are expected to contribute to the improvement of health in the society at large. The findings in this study sit well within previous research, which describes networks as vehicles or drivers of innovation that function inside the government (Considine, Lewis, & Alexander, 2009). Similarly, the network developed in the case of ÇPSSGP represents a case of innovation inside the government triggered by academic entrepreneurs in close cooperation with experts working in related government departments.

In addition, academic policy entrepreneurs contribute to evidence-based policy development, and eventually, methodological policy development, through sharing scientific research evidence and practices in the area of public health among several stakeholders. Despite this positive background, it is important to emphasize that evidence should inform all stages of policy making from policy formulation to policy implementation in order to contribute to policy learning. Otherwise, it risks turning into "solely technical exercise" (Sanderson, 2002, p. 19) confined to early stages of policy making without any real impact on final policy outcomes. Therefore, whether evidence-based policy making under ÇPSSGP will stimulate policy learning in the long run or remain a short-term experimentation remains a question mark. Overall, the achievements of the ÇPSSGP have been hold in high regard among policy practitioners who expect the same performance from stakeholders at the policy implementation stage (Özkan, 2018).

PPP Based Healthcare Construction Projects

Network Policy Background

PPPs are being used extensively in the areas of health service provision, health infrastructure, product development, and management of health facilities. PPP based projects are "a popular mode of tackling large, complicated, and expensive public health problems" (Reich, 2002, p. 62, p. vii), particularly in low- and middle-income countries, where governments lacking adequate financial, human, and technological resources embark on big-size projects and ambitious policy initiatives in partnership with private sector actors. A relatively new body of literature has developed concerning the role and effectiveness of PPPs in these countries including Turkey (Basu, Andrews, Kishore, Panjabi, & Stuckler, 2012; Chen & Feng, 2017; Campos, Norman, & Jadad, 2011; Kraak & Story, 2010; Murthy, Frieden, Yazdani, & Hreshikesh, 2001; Schwartz & Bhushan, 2004; Tekin & Çelik, 2010; Top & Sungur, 2019). From a governance perspective, PPPs have been expressed in "a myriad of other terms including but not limited to collaboration, alliance, coalition, network, inter-organizational relationship, joint advocacy campaign, and taskforce" (Johnston & Finegood, 2015, p. 257).

In the case of Turkey, PPP based projects represent a strategic policy instrument and investment method utilized by the MoH and triggered by the EU and WHO to facilitate the construction of healthy cities. Technically, PPP based projects are designed at the national level within the MoH with the General Directorate of Health Investments being the primarily responsible institution regarding policy planning and are applied at the local level based on a close partnership with private actors (i.e., big-size construction companies operating in Turkey). The purpose of such partnerships is to build huge integrated hospital campuses in some of the main cities in Turkey including Adana, Ankara, Bursa, Elaziğ, Eskişehir, Istanbul, Izmir, Kayseri, Konya, and Mersin.[9] Some of the main PPP based projects implemented are the following: Kayseri Integrated Health Campus (the first PPP project implemented in Turkey), Ankara Etlik Integrated Health Campus Project, Ankara Bilkent Integrated Health Campus Project, and Adana Integrated Health Campus Project. According to the information provided by the MoH during the interview process (expert working in the Health Investments Directorate), some of the main private companies involved in PPP based healthcare construction projects are YDA-Ronesans, Emsas – NKY, and Apco Meg. The PPP based model implemented in the Turkish healthcare sector is a build lease transfer (BLT) arrangement which applies to lengthy projects that can be extended up to 30 years. "The ultimate goal of the Ministry of Health is a total of 90,000 new beds throughout Turkey by the end of 2018" (McKenzie, 2015).[10]

The legal basis upon which PPP based projects operate has been subject to debate and controversy between two opposing camps in Turkey. The construction and renovation of integrated health facilities through the PPP based model constitutes a strategic policy goal, included within the HTP reform package introduced in 2003. However, the implementation of the project was delayed until the second

---

[9]More information on healthcare construction projects in Turkey can be found under the following links. Awarded contracts: https://sygm.saglik.gov.tr/TR,33960/sehir-hastaneleri.html; and construction tracking system http://yts.saglikyatirimlari.gov.tr/PublicYatirimlar.aspx?il=ANKARA.

[10]McKenzie (2015).

term of the ruling AK Party. Since 2009, the MoH has been actively involved in tendering and contract negotiation processes with various construction companies in Turkey. Despite the political will to get involved in such partnerships, PPP based projects faced legal challenges amid fierce opposition from political land societal elites. The implementation of the projects was temporarily suspended in 2012 by the Turkish Supreme Administrative Court (T.C. Danıştay Başkanlığı) and resumed with the enactment of the Law No. 6428 Concerning the Construction of Facilities, Renovation of Existing Facilities, and Purchasing Service by the MoH by PPP Model first enacted by the Turkish Parliament in 2013[11] and further amended in 2014.[12] According to this legal framework, PPPs are essentially common investment projects regulated by the provisions of the private law.

Previous studies have criticized PPP based healthcare construction projects in Turkey as another form of market enterprise which, contrary to expectations, is very expensive and ineffective and, most importantly, has no clear standards on how to achieve equity in healthcare services (Ataay, 2018; Öncü, 2017; Turkish Chamber of Engineers Architects, Ankara Office (TMMOB)/ Chamber of Medical Doctors, Ankara Office (ATO), 2017). In this study, PPP based projects are not approached as simply another investment opportunity for big construction companies. From a governance perspective, PPP based projects are essentially collaborative attempts that go beyond the interest of one or a group of companies and are expected to contribute to high quality health service delivery in Turkey by adapting modern healthcare standards. Field research reveals that such partnerships involve a cross-sectoral collaboration among stakeholders who interact in a repetitive fashion with the purpose of project development and management and produce tangible outcomes concerning health infrastructure and related services with a direct impact on the health of individual citizens. Over time, PPP based projects lead to a peculiar form of cross-sectoral collaboration, with dispersed cost and shared benefits as well as interdependence between the parties. Hence, in this study, PPP based projects qualify as a type of network collaboration involving primarily public actors and big construction companies operating in the healthcare construction sector. Without entering into a discussion of the benefits and drawbacks of the PPP based project outcomes for the health of individual citizens, the following sections provide an assessment of the factors that foster or inhibit this distinct form of network collaboration.

Network Structure

As mentioned above, PPP based healthcare construction projects comprise primarily state-business relations with the purpose of building and renovating hospital buildings and managing facility services. They can be considered as real estate projects with low levels of stakeholder involvement due to "fewer stakeholders present," less stakeholder interest "in participating in decision-making processes of

[11]http://www.resmigazete.gov.tr/eskiler/2013/03/20130309-1.htm
[12]http://www.resmigazete.gov.tr/eskiler/2014/05/20140509-26.htm

the projects," and lack of "stricter formal participation requirements" compared to other areas where PPP model is applied (Nederhand & Klijn, 2019, p. 1217). Similarly, PPP based healthcare construction projects in Turkey display low levels of actor inclusiveness in terms of type rather than number of actors involved, mainly due to the non-involvement of key NGOs and professional associations in the collaboration among public and private organizations. In the case of Turkey, this can be explained in part by the fact that professional associations such as TMMOB and ATO, among others, are diametrically opposed to the implementation of the PPP based healthcare construction projects.

Besides inclusiveness, another important aspect of network structure is connectedness. Actors engage in frequent interactions concerning ground level operations. Nonetheless, fewer interactions take place in the early stages of policy making, which remain highly centralized and hierarchical. The interviews reveal that the communication between network participants takes place occasionally in certain agreed days of the month. In addition, the interviewees mention that most of the interaction is not in the form of face-to-face communication but through formal inter-institutional communication. As a result, this type of network collaboration displays relatively low levels of connectedness among involved actors. PPP based network collaboration between public and private actors emerges at the operational stage of policy making (i.e., project implementation phase). During the implementation phase, long-term contracts of at least 10-year contracts regulate the behavior of stakeholders in a way that each actor has clear responsibilities from the onset of the project. Certainly, sharing investment responsibilities entails continuous cost and benefit calculations from all stakeholders who might be faced with unanticipated challenges that require strategic decision-making. However, this is an exception to the rule. Naturally, PPP based healthcare construction projects in Turkey record only minimal levels of common decision-making (0.20/1.00).

In Turkey, PPP based healthcare construction projects are applied in areas characterized by high costs and eventually high risks. The glue that brings actors together in such lengthy and costly projects consists of sharing tangible resources (e.g., material, technological, or financial resources) as well as knowledge based resources (e.g., information or expertise), contributing to high levels of resource pooling which in turn leads to high levels of interdependence among network participants. PPP based projects involve strict job division concerning day-to-day operations. Public actors are primarily responsible for project planning at the early stages of policy making and project evaluation at the latter stages of policy making. Both public and private actors are equally responsible for project development and management throughout the collaboration process. Private companies are responsible for the construction of health campuses and for the management of the hospitals for a specified number of years after the buildings are ready for use. Public actors are primarily responsible for financing the projects and for the recruitment of doctors, nurses, and technicians after the construction period is over. However, they rely on the technical expertise and experience of the private companies in the field of healthcare construction and facility management. Following this logic, it would be accurate to say that PPP based projects are benefit sharing (i.e., interaction is contingent upon lowering risks though the division of responsibilities) rather than profit driven at least not in the strict sense where interaction is contingent upon maximizing returns. PPP based projects operate through collaborative networks where all actors are expected to generate a win–win situation that aims at reducing investment risks.

The presence of long-term contracting entails that this policy network is highly regularized. Regulations include both *ex ante* and *ex post* rules that ensure the enforcement of the contract in the context of long-term capital deployment. According to the information retrieved from the MoH, punishment measures were taken very rarely, consisting only in 10% of the cases. Such a low score shows that the terms of the contract, agreed at the inception of the collaboration, are rarely broken during the implementation stage. Yet, the public sector representatives admit that long-term contracting involves many challenges associated with management and enforcement which can be overcome through already established mechanisms of dispute resolution comparable to developed countries with extended experience in PPP application such as the UK.[13] Overall, high levels of resource pooling as well as presence of binding rules and enforcement regulation contribute to high levels of interdependence at the network level (0.87/1).

Despite having a highly interdependent structure, PPP based policy networks do not have the necessary mechanisms for negotiating substantive issues or critical decision-making issues among parties (low levels of horizontal coordination). There is a perception among public organization representatives that they have the upper hand in project planning and management, whereas private actors are ultimately accountable to the state. This argument is confirmed by governmental reports where "PPP based model represents an asymmetric situation that is in favour of the public administration"[14] (Ministry of Development, 2017). Hence, a perception of equal bargaining power is missing leading to low levels of horizontal coordination among network participants.

Overall, in spite of high levels of interdependence largely lacking mechanisms of common decision-making and horizontal coordination coupled with low levels of connectedness among actors all contribute to low levels of network structural capacity (0.37/1.00). In the absence of equal bargaining and common decision-making mechanisms, intra-network interactions are regulated by enforcement mechanisms that are specified in the contract in the form of rules of procedure. In such cases, strict contract enforcement and effective network management serve as a substitute for loose network ties which bond network participants under an overarching goal and make interaction possible on a daily basis within the framework of long-term project implementation.

[13]For more information on the Turkish experience in dispute resolution concerning PPPs, see Skilling (2015).

[14]Translated from Turkish to English by the author. The original version is "İşbirliği modelinde, kamu yönetimi lehine asimetrik bir durum da söz konusudur." Ministry of Development (2017).

Intra-network Ties

As mentioned above, network interaction in PPPs takes the form of strict contract enforcement of various dispersed institutions that work in a quasi-autonomous fashion through strict job division which does not require much face-to-face contact. Hence, trust is not an issue in PPP based networks. Naturally, this type of network collaboration exhibits relatively low scores of trust-based interactions at the network level. Clearly, companies with some credibility in the government are selected in the tendering process. Hence, there is some level of inter-organizational trust manifested in the form of willingness to cooperate, goal convergence, and some team work among a limited number of actors in high levels of decision-making which does not convert into a synergetic type of team work concerning daily activities.

Even though presence of trust is highly improbable within this collaborative setting, interviewees highlight the importance of a collaborative spirit among stakeholders. According to an interview with a public sector representative, PPP based projects should be based on a synergic model where the parties must act as a whole (e.g., high-level bureaucrats working in the Health Investments Directorate). In addition, the insistence of public actors on establishing a management team as soon as possible to administer day-to-day operational challenges implies that close, trust-based relations between the parties are missing. Overall, PPP based collaborative networks display a low score of inter-organizational level trust and no inter-personal level trust. Lack of inter-personal trust can be partially explained by the nature of collaboration (i.e., strictly formal relations regulated by terms and conditions of the contract), and partially by the lack of frequent, face-to-face communication between network participants throughout the collaboration process.

Network Institutionalization

PPP based healthcare construction investments are on-going projects with concrete policy outcomes. Despite having a weak internal structure and weak ties among parties, healthcare construction projects are still running in Turkey currently and yielding policy outcomes in the field of healthcare construction. Persistence of these projects despite the changing political environment and economic conditions is a clear evidence of the institutional resilience of this type of network collaboration. Presence of a global discourse in favor of PPP based projects in low- and middle-income countries, presence of a domestic policy agenda on the issue of healthcare construction, political willingness to implement the projects despite legal obstacles and political opposition, existing alliance between the government, and big-size corporations in the construction sector are some factors that account for high levels of institutional resilience in the context of PPPs. PPP based healthcare construction projects have been among the most publicized items in the agenda of the ruling AK Party since their second ruling term (since 2009). These projects have gained political and economic prominence for various reasons. Construction of healthy cities is a grand project promoted by the WHO and at the same time a globally spread movement which aims at increasing the health standards of many cities in the world through urban lifestyle transformation. On the other side, and more importantly, PPP projects fit into the AK Party governing agenda which prioritizes hospital centered services as key to health policy development in Turkey. Last but not least, AKP has built strong and durable alliances with capital factions in the construction sector – a situation that has been covered extensively by scholars as a driving force behind Turkish politics in the recent years (Demiralp, 2018; Karatepe, 2016; Ocaklı, 2018; Öniş, 2019). Such alliances have been critical for the institutional resilience of PPPs in Turkey.

In addition, PPPs are based upon a legal framework that impedes third party attempts to sue or annul the projects. Legal provisions introduced in 2013 were attempt to curtail if not eliminate the administrative and bureaucratic control on PPPs. Since then, the contracts that regulate PPPs have been subject to private law rather than public administrative court revisions. Besides legal arrangements, a separate government department specialized in PPP operations has already been established under the MoH, the General Directorate of Investments. The interviews reveal that the PPP model is constantly being revised and refined by experts working in this institution. Considering all the above, network collaboration in the area of healthcare construction exhibits an exceptionally high score of institutionalization (1.00/1.00). To sum up, PPP based partnerships represent an institutionally resilient network arrangement. From the governance perspective, they constitute an effective model of network collaboration that crosses the divides between the state and the businesses within the Turkish health policy sector and reconfigures the roles and responsibilities of these actors in health policy development.

Network Policy Impact

Overall, PPP based partnerships constitute a network type of collaboration characterized by relatively low levels of structural and relational capacity and high levels of institutional capacity at the network level as defined in this study. Despite having a fragile network structure and weak intra-network ties, PPP based investment projects are deeply embedded in the surrounding political and economic environment receiving high levels of political and financial support, particularly from the central government. In addition, they are built upon a supportive legal framework and solid business-based alliance which account for the on-going collaboration with concrete policy outcomes.

From a comparative perspective, PPP based projects are presented as hybrid types which stand in between network governance and neo-corporate governance, or, stated differently, between policy networks and subcontracting. Even though PPPs are in vogue there is an ongoing language game concerning this concept (Hodge & Greve, 2007). According to Stephen Wilks (2013) partnerships can best be described as "a mutual understanding between political and corporate leaders which … can be creatively and accurately analyzed through the lenses of elitism" (p. 41) without the need for more pluralist approaches to governance. There is some truth in this statement. However, this line of thinking does not account for management of collaboration on daily basis as well as the outcomes of PPPs which are expected to go beyond the self-interested goals of corporations and increase the quality of public services toward citizens. Despite being based on a strong business alliance, this interaction does not fall under the category of corporate governance *strictu sensu*. PPP based projects in middle- and low-income countries are as flexible alliances with the purpose of carrying out big investment projects (i.e., network analysis), rather than stable, organic links between government and businesses upon which the whole political system is based (i.e., neo-corporatist model). One way to approach PPPs through the lenses of network analysis would be through the concept of "heterogeneous policy networks," where involved actors mediate their interests and exchange their resources (Börzel, 1997).

Moreover, PPP based projects should not considered as another case of subcontracting. In this study, PPP based collaborative networks display a degree of common decision-making and high levels of interdependence among involved parties. Projects based on the method of subcontracting are characterized by asymmetrical power distribution, centralized control, and explicit resource dependence on the state. These are closed networks accessed by only some non-governmental or private actors chosen arbitrarily by the state for the purpose of outsourcing. The state here serves as the leading force, chief architect, funder, coordinator, and center of authority. Subcontracting might represent a new form of governance but a traditional logic of governing (e.g., hierarchical) which contradicts the very essence of network collaboration. Considering that subcontracted organizations depend completely on external resources one could also use the lenses of resource dependency theory to explain such practices of policy implementation.

In this study, PPPs represent a form of network collaboration which turns out to be effective in the context of high-risk, capital-intensive, and long-term projects. More than anything else, PPP based network collaboration shows that collaboration can be durable as long as it is effective in terms of achieving anticipated policy outcomes. In the Turkish case, policy effectiveness can be attributed to, among others, the institutional embeddedness of networks into the broader political and economic environment, particularly the support received by already existing business alliances which contribute to the institutional resilience of these policy networks. This example shows that networks that serve as channels of interest intermediation are highly resilient and effective policy instruments. In more concrete terms, PPP based projects contribute to better health services through renewed infrastructure and technical expertise in the construction and management of the health facilities. Moreover, such projects are expected to foster cooperation between public and private actors through benefit sharing and risk reduction in a policy sub-area of scarce resources. Finally, such projects stimulate private actors contribute to public policy goals. If such projects are not only one-sided investment opportunities for profit maximization, they help the companies to engage in the implementation of national health policy strategies and develop corporate social responsibility.

Two potential problems can emerge in this type of collaborative arrangement. Both of these problems are linked to the issue of long-term management of collaboration.[15] First, important decisions are taken early in the policy making process by high level bureaucrats in the ministerial departments. In time, such collaborative arrangements may turn into hierarchical structures that lose their collaborative spirit. A second problem is that of network productiveness in the long run. Despite strict job division, the absence of an effective management team might prompt the actors to work toward their own specific goals rather than collective goals giving rise to conflict of interest problems. This situation might diminish the productiveness of network participants in the long run especially after the construction of health facilities. Therefore, the long-term applicability of the PPP based project depends on the effective use of contract enforcement mechanisms as well as incentives that would enhance credibility between parties (see Bertelli & Smith, 2009). As it has been emphasized in previous studies, more than anything else the effectiveness of PPP based projects is a function of good management (Tekin & Çelik, 2010). Good management on the other hand is very much a function of:

> the effective use of expertise on the side of the selected private companies and the willingness of all parties to embrace a "spirit of partnership" based on a framework of transparency, fairness and equality. (KOI 2019–2023 Report, p. 40)

Health Tourism Coordination Council (SATURK)

Network Policy Background

One of the most recent trends in the healthcare sector is the globalization of health services. Globalization refers to the patient movement beyond national borders to benefit from health services of other countries, widely discussed in the literature as health tourism. Advanced industrialized countries such as Germany, Singapore, Switzerland, UK and the USA have long been actors of global health tourism. However, recently, the reputation of countries such as Hungary, India, Macedonia, Malaysia, Malta, Thailand, and Turkey is growing rapidly due to relatively lower prices coupled by increasing quality of the healthcare services. In Turkey, health tourism sector is expanding and prospering enormously with a growing number of accredited health centers receiving patients from all over the world. In the last 10 years, the government in Turkey has prioritized health tourism development with the assumption that it has positive spill overs for the economic development of Turkey, and it serves as a soft policy instrument improving the image of Turkey abroad.

---

[15]Public management is a recurring theme in network analysis. Below are some important overview works that deal with the issue: Agranoff (2006), Agranoff and McGuire (1999, 2001), Agranoff and Yıldız (2007), Kickert and Koppenjan (1997), and McGuire and Agranoff (2011).

Policy making in the area of health tourism covers a vast number of actors from different sectors (i.e., public, private, and voluntary) as well as different policy domains, such as health, tourism, culture, and economy. The main public institution responsible for the development of health tourism strategy at the national level is the MoH, the General Directorate of Health Services, and the Department of Health Tourism established in 2011.[16] Health tourism is both a national policy priority and a regional development goal. Thus, network collaboration within this policy sub-area requires multiple stakeholders including government representatives from the central and local levels, private business representatives, and professional associations both at the national and regional levels. Overall, considering the large number of involved actors at the national, regional, and local level of policy making, health tourism as a policy sub-area represents a fertile ground for the formation of policy networks.

Enhanced health tourism has been announced as one of the MoH's strategic goals published in 2012 which aims "to continue to develop the health system as a means to contributing to the economic and social development of Turkey and to global health"[17] (Ministry of Health, Strategic Plan, p. 18). To this end, one of the policy objectives of the MoH is to improve health tourism governance. In this context, the MoH aims:

> To establish scientific counseling boards to ensure that health tourism practices are carried out as evidence-based. To continue the cooperation with the sectors on investment, planning and incentives within the framework of health tourism. To cooperate with the other sectors to identify the education standards for the intermediary/support staff to work in health tourism services and to provide their education in cooperation with the Ministry of Education and the Council of Higher Education .... To cooperate with the national and international professional organizations, NGO's and the private sector. (Ministry of Health, Strategic Plan, pp. 119–120)

Policy collaboration in the area of health tourism was elaborated in a more detailed fashion in the Health Tourism Development Program in 2013. The program coordinated by the MoH and the Ministry of Culture and Tourism among others aimed at "developing coordination mechanisms between public institutions, strengthening the cooperation between public and private sectors" in building a legal infrastructure for health tourism and "increasing the collaborations of public and private sectors in advertising and marketing" (MoH, 2013, p. 8) health tourism.[18]

---

[16]Health Tourism Department running under the General Directorate of Health Promotion (2011–2016); the General Directorate of Health Services (since 2016).
[17]Ministry of Health (2012).
[18]Ministry of Health (2013).

Cross-sectoral collaboration in the field of health tourism has reached its pinnacle with the establishment of the Health Tourism Coordination Council (SATURK). SATURK was established in 2015 after a series of cross-sectoral encounters among stakeholders from the public, private and voluntary sectors. SATURK is an inter-agency coordination council composed of various organizations that are responsible for different aspects of health tourism development, such as the MoH, Ministry of Culture and Tourism, Ministry of Economy, Ministry of Family and Social Policy, Ministry of Development, Ministry of Labour and Social Security, representatives from representatives from the Council of Higher Education (YÖK), the Union of Chambers and Commodity Exchanges of Turkey (TOBB), the Foreign Economic Relations Board (DEİK), and the Turkish Cooperation and Coordination Agency (TİKA), who are expected to represent the interests of all the stakeholders within the health tourism sector. When first established in 2015, Prime Minister's Office held the leadership position of the Council (Government Circular, 2015/3).[19]

SATURK supervises three work groups: (1) Advertising and Pricing Commission, (2) Education and Planning Commission, and (3) The Regulations and Accreditation Commission. These are joint work groups composed of actors from the public, private, and voluntary sectors. Many service delivery institutions within the field of health tourism work under the supervision of SATURK including healthcare suppliers, insurance companies, hotel and hospitality enterprises, travel agencies, tourist information centers, and logistics firms. Stakeholders are jointly responsible for building business relations with other countries on the issue of health tourism, planning and coordinating the movement of foreign patients to Turkey, and preparing the ground for patient hospitalization in health facilities in Turkey.

Network Structure

Considering the number and the type of organizations involved, SATURK supervises an inclusive, multi-actor, and multi-tiered policy network that links decision-makers at the national level with practitioners and service providers at the local level. The policy network operating under SATURK displays high levels of actor inclusiveness (0.80/1.00) both in terms of number (network size) and also type of actors (network heterogeneity). SATURK is the broadest policy network compared to other cases under investigation including governmental organizations (i.e., central and local level), private sector representatives, NGOs, and professional associations operating within the field of health tourism. Considering the number and types of actors involved, SATURK is responsible for coordinating intra-governmental relations (i.e., multiple ministerial departments and offices at different levels of government), government-NGO relations (i.e., multiple NGOs and professional associations operating in the field of health tourism), and government business relations (i.e., private sector representatives).

[19]Official Gazette, 7 Şubat 2015, No. 29260: http://www.saturk.gov.tr/images/pdf/genelge.pdf.

The biggest challenge of such an inclusive and complex network is the alignment of several actors within a functioning structure which, among others, requires continuing interaction among network participants. A functioning network requires high levels of actor connectedness in the form of vertical integration among actors at different levels of governance and horizontal coordination among ministerial departments within the central government as well as logistical organizations and service providers operating in the field. Despite the need for continuing interaction, SATURK displays average levels of connectedness among actors. Interviewees reveal that multi-stakeholder meetings have been constantly interrupted and postponed due to events such as the general election campaigns or political and institutional transformations. Furthermore, communication among different organizational representatives has been carried out mainly through internet and/or phone channels rather than through direct, face-to-face channels of communication which can negatively influence network level connectedness. Overall, SATURK displays a medium score of network level connectedness, which indicates that channels of communication are not at expected levels considering the complexity of the network type under consideration.

Found between the policy design and policy implementation stage, SATURK has been established at a certain phase of the policy making cycle where critical decision that ensure policy coherence need to be taken. Content analysis reveals that SATURK scores particularly low in terms of common decision-making (0.20/1.00). Even though multi-stakeholder meetings are held, decision-making is concentrated within the ministerial cabinet, particularly taking the form of correspondence between the MoH and the Prime Minister's Office. In addition, the MoH with its role as the secretariat of SATURK prepares and finalizes the policy alternatives. Metaphorically, the ministerial departments cook the decisions in their own kitchen without much input from other actors. Practically, multi-stakeholder meetings provide only limited space for common decision-making.

SATURK also displays a relatively low score of actor interdependence (0.37/1.00) which can be explained by low levels of resource pooling. Network collaboration taking place under SATURK does not involve exchange of material resources and/or exchange of expertise. Multi-stakeholder meetings take the form of broad deliberative platforms which are essentially consultative in nature and do not generate binding decisions. The advantage of these platforms is that they facilitate the regular exchange of ideas among different stakeholders through cross-sectoral deliberations. They do not involve systematic exchange of expertise translatable to policy making. One of the interviewees illustrate this point by arguing that unless such meetings turn into platforms of knowledge exchange, they will remain shallow/empty meetings that host large numbers of attendants yet not participants (DEIK representative). Concerning horizontal coordination, SATURK displays a relatively low score (0.20/1.00). As mentioned above, interaction within multi-stakeholder meetings takes the form of deliberation with limited space for exercise of power. Within this type of setting, network participants have a limited perception of equal influence on policy decisions. They are well aware that substantive issues are not negotiated and even open to debate.

Interviews reveal that the dynamics behind SATURK is more complex than it seems. Critical decisions are taken within a core group of actors, including high level bureaucrats working within the MoH, the General Directorate of Health Promotion, and the Directorate of Health Tourism (at the time of interview) together with individuals from selected NGOs with experience in project management both within the government and in the field of health tourism.[20] Due to their connections with public sector officials, these NGOs can penetrate the black box of decision-making within the MoH by influencing high level bureaucrats. At the same time, these NGOs serve as a bridge between decision-makers within the central government and multiple service providers operating in the ground at the pre-operational stage of policy making. In more concrete terms, NGO representatives engage in constant consultations with high level officials and other public authorities (i.e., commission meetings and semi-informal meetings), transfer information to service providers and professional associations concerning issues such as medical tourism marketing strategy, accreditation, and certification, and offer logistical support on the ground (e.g., consultancy on medical and travel services, organizational services).

At a more theoretical level, these NGOs serve as brokers or intermediaries who facilitate "organizational-knowledge-sharing," a concept elaborated within organizational studies (Cabrera & Cabrera, 2002; Chow & Chan, 2008; Kim & Lee, 2006; Van Den Hooff & De Ridder, 2004). Here, organizational-knowledge-sharing does not refer to sharing technical expertise by professionals of a similar background within small, semi-formal work groups like the ÇPSSGP case nor does it refer to sharing project output information by organizations within a formal structure regulated by contract enforcement as in the PPP case. In this instance, organizational-knowledge-sharing refers sharing governmental decisions that guide the course of action on the ground or procedures that need to be followed by a large community of actors operating within the field of health tourism. Following this logic, NGOs working closely with public offices within the central government facilitate organizational-knowledge-sharing within the multi-tier network structure formed under SATURK.

Organizational knowledge-sharing is the key to a functioning multi-tier network structure such as SATURK. However, having a limited number of NGOs or a single NGO carrying out the function of the intermediary within a broad network of actors is a temporary fix rather than a permanent solution. Building a mechanism that facilitates systematic and continuous knowledge-sharing among organizations, such as the development of an information technology (IT) system accessed by all organizations, is key to the effectiveness of Commissions operating under SATURK in addition to the long-term network collaboration in the field of health tourism. Previous research has found that "usage of IT applications are all positively associated with high levels of employee knowledge-sharing

[20]Sağlık Turizmi Geliştirme Destekleme Ve Organizasyon Hizmetleri Derneği is one of the NGOs specialized in health tourism promotion, support and organizational services, which works in close partnership to the government.

capabilities" (Kim & Lee, 2006, p. 370). Another drawback of having such a core group within the broad network structure is that the cross-sectoral collaboration can in time dissolve leading the way to cooperation between few actors that are not representative of the respective policy area. This NGO plays the role of a subcontracted organization or a government run organization. Under such circumstances, the government may change the subcontracted NGOs frequently based on the quality of the service provision. This will prompt the marketization of the non-profit service providers (Eikenberry & Kluver, 2004) in the field of health tourism which runs contrary to the logic of network governance built upon a symmetrical and reciprocal structure of relatively stable relations among stakeholders.

Overall, high levels of actor inclusiveness turn out to be both a blessing and a curse for policy network operating under SATURK. In one regard, SATURK is a broad policy network with representatives from all the policy sectors (i.e., public, private, and voluntary) a relatively open space that facilitates exchange of ideas between various actors through deliberation at the cross-sectoral level. Yet, on the other hand, this policy network largely lacks common decision-making mechanisms as well as reciprocity mechanisms including benefit sharing, enforcement, and equal bargaining mechanisms that bond network participants together within a truly collaborative structure. Therefore, currently SATURK exhibits low levels of structural capacity which can be strengthened by developing a system of organizational-knowledge-sharing that will bond public, private, and voluntary actors operating in the field of health tourism within a functioning multi-tier network structure.

Intra-network Ties

The policy network operating under SATURK displays an average score (0.5/1.00) in terms of its capacity to maintain intra-network ties through trust-based interaction (relational capacity). This network consists of a representative and broad constellation of actors, comprising of public, private, and voluntary sectors, gathered around an umbrella issue (i.e., enhanced health tourism). Multi-stakeholder meetings leading to the formation of SATURK take the form of aggregate rather than integrated platforms. Thus, the policy network established within the area of health tourism consists of a loose web of actors which makes the development of inter-organizational trust in the form of synergetic team work hardly possible. In more concrete terms, content analysis reveals some degree of inter-organizational level trust built upon the willingness of various organization to come together and cooperate on common goals concerning health tourism development which does not go beyond a general sense of solidarity. Synergy observed in the work groups operating under ÇPSSGP was absent from multi-stakeholder meetings that led to the formation of SATURK. It is possible though that trust levels will increase over time if network participants get closer through regular team work collaboration.

Moreover, inter-personal trust is present only among some NGO representatives and high-level officials involved in decision-making within the core group which operates within the MoH. Overall, lack of adequate structure that facilitates collaboration among a large group of stakeholders coupled with average levels of trust might lead to collective action problems in the medium and long terms.

Network Institutionalization

The policy developed under SATURK exhibits average levels of network institutionalization (0.62/1.00). SATURK receives necessary political support from prominent political leaders and high-level state officials responsible for the development of health tourism at the national level. Health tourism development as a strategic policy goal has been ranked very high on the political agenda of the ruling AK Party. Moreover, since 2011, a ministerial department within the central government has been established responsible primarily for "carr[ying] out operations and procedures related to health tourism in coordination with related institutions and organizations" (General Directorate of Health Tourism).[21] Contrary to these institutional achievements, neither a business alliance between private actors nor a broad coalition between government representatives and private sector representatives has been developed. The establishment of SATURK itself as an inter-agency institutional arrangement that promotes policy coordination and adds to the overall institutionalization of collaboration within the field of health tourism.

Even though this study offers some insights, institutionalization of network collaboration within the policy sub-area of health tourism in Turkey should be subject to further research. The strength of this network stands in the presence of strong political support from high level officials and the establishment of formal institutions within the government contributing to network institutionalization. Yet, its weakness stands in the lack of legal agreement between parties, lack of a long-term integration strategy that coordinates all actors on the ground, and the risk of changing political priorities that might lead to network dissolution. Moreover, at the time of the interview, SATURK and its related commissions had not yet entered the policy implementation stage. As a result, institutional resilience of the policy network under investigation has not yet been put to test.

Network Policy Impact

As mentioned above, the policy network supervised by the Health Tourism Council (SATURK) takes the form of aggregate actor constellation. On the one hand, this network is highly heterogeneous in terms of number of stakeholders representing a variety of interests, preferences, and motivations (i.e., high levels of differentiation). On the other hand, this network lacks enough mechanisms to bond these stakeholders within a structure of continuous exchange and common decision-making. Hence, the true challenge here stands in aligning actors from

---

[21]https://sagliktu rizmi.saglik.gov.tr/EN,24507/duties-of-our-presidency.html

different sectors and levels of governance within a functioning network structure. Cross-sectoral collaboration at the policy design stage is made possible through encounters among stakeholders in the form of large deliberative fora (i.e., issue network) and a small core group of actors at the center which accelerated decision-making processes. Currently, the establishment of SATURK represents a more advanced stage of network collaboration within the area of health tourism at the stage between policy formulation and policy implementation.

Structurally, the network in the field of health tourism represents an issue network as defined by Rhodes in his analysis of the British policy environment. Issue networks often serve as venues to raise awareness around an issue, develop a policy agenda, promote a shared policy vision, or develop a common policy strategy. Such networks are particularly important for promoting cross-sectoral deliberation and developing common strategies at the early stages of policy making. However, issue networks are composed of actors from different policy sectors who are loosely connected to each other. As the name indicates, what brings these actors together is the umbrella issue under which they operate. Umbrella issue networks are built upon heterogeneous webs of relationships which can hardly become well-integrated structures of collaborative policy making. Another notably similar network category is that introduced by Niamh Hardiman (2006) in his analysis of flexible network governance. Hardiman describes Irish policy networks as social partnerships centered around policy issues not contained to one strict policy area. Social partnerships incorporate diverse actors such as "civil servants as well as ... unions, employers, and representatives of the community sector of voluntary organizations, advocacy groups, and special interest bodies with some form of statutory basis" (Hardiman, 2006, p. 344). Policy networks, according to Hardiman (2006), are very dynamic, fluid, and diffuse structures. Similar to the network operating under SATURK, the "ultimate decisions in 'flexible network governance' rest with the government" (p. 348). This type of network collaboration can be considered truly cross-sectoral; a type of interaction where actor coordination becomes a significantly challenging task (Herranz, 2007).

Even though the structure of SATURK is diffuse, close, and continuous interaction between key government officials and selected NGO representatives, as in the case of the core group mentioned above accelerates decision-making and pushes network collaboration forward. The current collaboration between governmental and non-governmental actors in the field of health tourism takes place primarily in order to carry out logistical tasks that cannot be accomplished by public actors on the ground and coordination tasks that reduce the transaction costs among numerous actors through organizational-knowledge-sharing. However, the informal alliance between government officials and NGO representatives has a temporary nature. Organizational knowledge-sharing can be institutionalized through IT information applications and incorporated within the workings of the Commissions under the formal structure of SATURK.

Despite future risks and possibilities, currently SATURK is an inter-agency arrangement which serves as a coordination mechanism between various ministerial department as well as a bridge between decision-making at the national level and policy implementation at the local level. The establishment of SATURK is a manifestation of an inclusive and holistic approach to policy making in the area of health tourism in Turkey. Even though some degree of policy coherence has been achieved at the pre-operational stage, the interviews carried out in 2015 reveal that there are no clear guidelines on how to carry out cross-sectoral collaboration at the policy implementation stage. The future success of this type of collaboration is contingent upon an effective organizational-knowledge-sharing which takes places at three levels of governance: (a) inter-agency coordination among various ministerial departments following an all-of-government approach; (b) vertical integration between government representatives, private sector representatives, NGOs, and service providers with the purpose of policy coherence; and (c) horizontal coordination among service providers, logistical organizations, and various other organizations operating in the field of health tourism. To sum up, the effectiveness of this type of network collaboration depends upon achieving a cohesive policy framework which facilitates integration among various actors operating across different policy fields and different levels of governance.

Conclusion

This study offers a minimal and parsimonious definition of policy networks as platforms that facilitate cross-sectoral interaction which takes place in a repetitive and regular fashion and has some measurable policy impact. The main assumption here is that networks are not inherently collaborative as it is often assumed in the literature. Each network demonstrates a varying capacity to collaborate contingent upon factors internal and external to network structure that should be measured empirically. This chapter develops a new measure used to assess NCC through structural, relational, and institutional factors that influence network collaboration. This measure has been applied in the context of cross-sectoral collaboration that takes place with the purpose of health policy making in Turkey focusing in the period from 2011 to 2015. This chapter draws attention to variation in network collaboration through a detailed account of three networks in the policy sub-areas of public health policy development, healthcare investment, and health tourism.

The presence of cross-sectoral collaboration shows that policy networks are relevant instruments of policy making within the Turkish health sector which contradicts the idea that policy networks are completely lacking or go as far as being an imaginary phenomenon with no concrete policy implications. Overall, networks under consideration exhibit similar levels of overall NCC equal to 0.66 (ÇPSSGP), 0.59 (PPP), and 0.49 (SATURK). In more concrete terms, various stakeholders do have some capacity to interact in a collaborative fashion toward achieving certain policy goals with ÇPSSGP leading the list. However, overall collaborative capacity does not automatically translate into network effectiveness or persistence. Results of content analysis reveal that policy networks diverge in terms of their structural, relational, and institutional capacity to collaborate. Hence, it is not possible to talk about a monolithic and uniform concept or a single practice of network collaboration even at the sub-sectoral level. Instead, policy networks are flexible and continuously changing patterns that are expected to move along the continuum of collaborative capacity.

Among the three policy networks under investigation, collaboration under ÇPSSGP represents a case of very high levels of actor connectedness, horizontal coordination, and trust manifested in the form of willingness to cooperate, goal convergence, team work, synergy, and inter-personal trust, yet low levels of institutionalization. These results show that regardless of having a robust internal network dynamic, ÇPSSGP is not adequately entrenched in the external political and economic environment. Even though this network displays a robust internal structure through a successful government–university partnership and contributes to innovation in public health through the adoption of evidence-based approach to policy making, cross-sectoral collaboration is currently at a limbo state largely due to the lack of political willingness to push the program forward to the policy implementation stage.

PPP based co-investment projects represent a case of network collaboration diametrically opposed to the ÇPSSGP case with a fragile internal structure that displays very low levels of common decision-making and horizontal coordination and no synergetic team work among actors who operate in an autonomous fashion on the ground regulated by strict contract enforcement. Despite having weak intra-network ties and a loose collaborative structure, PPPs exhibit high levels of network institutionalization through legislation and formal institutions, which ensure smooth transition from policy formulation to policy implementation stage. PPPs represent a contractor-led approach to policy making generate better performing projects in the area of healthcare construction and ultimately results in higher quality public services for citizens, as long as they maintain the collaborative momentum among government and businesses and do not give rise to conflicts of interest.

Network collaboration taking place under the umbrella of SATURK displays very high levels of actor inclusiveness within a multi-tier network structure. However, this network displays particularly low levels of common decision-making, actor interdependence, horizontal coordination, and synergetic team work which suggest low levels of integration among a broad range of actors. Even though this network displays average levels of institutionalization, policy implementation has been postponed with no clear coordinates for cross-sectoral collaboration at the operational stage. Even though actor integration has not yet been achieved, SATURK represents an inclusive approach to policy making which expands the policy space in the area of health tourism and contributes to organizational-knowledge-sharing primarily through NGO–government partnership. Overall, network collaboration within the area of health tourism suggests that average levels of relational and institutional capacity can generate some degree of policy coherence though actor coordination and organizational-knowledge-sharing.

This chapter suggests that, among all others, institutionalization is a crucial aspect that not only maintains the collaborative momentum but is also capable for either sustaining or blocking interaction within the policy network altogether. Certainly, network collaboration has a structural and relational dimension which should be considered to assess and further strengthen NCC. However, institutionalization, or network embeddedness in the external environment, which provides the network with necessary political and economic support, seems to have a direct impact on the persistence and effectiveness of collaboration. The case of ÇPSSGP which fails to achieve policy effectiveness despite having a robust collaborative structure and strong intra-network ties illustrates best this case. Contrary to this case, PPPs do achieve policy outcomes with an impact on the health of individual citizens, regardless of having a fragile collaborative structure and loose intra-network ties. The effectiveness of PPPs can be attributed to high levels of institutional resilience of this type of collaboration which is entrenched in a solid alliance between government and businesses in the construction sector in Turkey. Consequently, future studies should pay more attention to network institutionalization especially in the form of network embeddedness in the surrounding external environment.

Finally, this chapter suggests that policy networks become significant policy instruments only when they are associated with some concrete policy impact. The cases under investigation show that policy networks can (a) turn into vehicles that diffuse policy innovation through intensive expertise sharing between government officials and university researchers, especially in the area of public health policy development, where academic entrepreneurs contribute to public policy formation (the ÇPSSGP case); (b) lower the risk of huge investment projects through contract based enforcement, especially in the policy area of healthcare investments, where the government and businesses share financial, technical, and human resources during the policy implementation stage (the PPP case); and (c) serve the purpose of organizational-knowledge-sharing among a broad range of actors, especially in the policy area of health tourism, though close NGO–government partnership at the pre-operational phase of policy making (i.e., the SATURK case). Despite some deficiencies, existing policy networks serve as opportunities that should not be squandered and should be developed by further strengthening their structural, relational, and institutional capacities.

Chapter 5

Tackling the Root Causes: Inherited Structural and Cultural Barriers to Policy Collaboration in Turkey

Abstract

While Chapter 3 highlights contextual conditions that foster the formation of policy networks, Chapter 5 highlights contextual conditions that impede the formation of policy networks. The overarching question of this chapter is the following: What are the factors that hinder cross-sectoral arrangements from becoming collaborative in complex policy settings such as low- and middle-income countries with a tradition in centralized policy making? In an attempt to address this question, this study provides a detailed assessment of all cross-sectoral arrangements within the Turkish health sector focusing on the post-2003 period. Within this framework, three types of networks will be examined including (a) consultative networks where stakeholders come together primarily to legitimize certain government policies within national level health policy platforms; (b) cluster networks where stakeholder interaction falls short of becoming collaborative due to diverging interests and persistent competition at the regional level; and (c) patronage networks where governmental actors and a selected number of NGOs linked by clientelism serve as a bridge between the ruling party and its constituency at the community level. Unlike policy networks, these actor constellations observed at different levels of governance do not serve the purpose of policy collaboration. On the contrary, they have the potential to trigger politicization, fragmentation, and even polarization at the social level, especially through the distribution of selective benefits. Ultimately, this chapter aims to rise to the challenge of policy collaboration by assessing the impediments to network collaboration based on insights from the Turkish case.

Keywords: Consultative networks; cluster networks; cross-sectoral collaboration; patronage networks; political culture; structural barriers

---

Network Policy Making within the Turkish Health Sector: Becoming Collaborative, 95–111

doi:10.1108/978-1-83867-094-820201006

> [...] the management of inter-organisational collaboration seems to be a challenge for practitioners as well as researchers in the field of public health. (Axelsson & Axelsson, 2006, p. 86)

Bringing stakeholders together with the purpose of collaboration in the area of public health is a challenge (Axelsson & Axelsson, 2006). "One of the main challenges is to bring ... organizations from different sectors together in a common pursuit of public health" (Axelsson & Axelsson, 2006, p. 76). The challenge here is less about organizational differences in terms of "formal structure of organizations" and more about "differences in values and cultures that are the most difficult barriers to integration" (Axelsson & Axelsson, 2006, p. 83) between organizations. The challenge is amplified in low- and middle-income country settings which are faced with several structural barriers to multi-sectoral action such as "lack of capacity, lack of resources, poor governance, corruption and weak accountability" (Rasanathan, Atkins, Mwansambo, Soucat, & Bennett, 2018, p. 4) coupled with a "high degree of internal fragmentation" (Bennett, Glandon, & Rasanathan, 2018, p. 3) within the health sector between organizations "along geographic and programme lines" (Bennett et al., 2018). Considering various challenges and opportunities existing in low- and middle-income countries, many studies have investigated the governance of multi-sectoral action and policy collaboration in these settings with a special attention given to the health sector as an increasingly complex policy environment (Abimbola, Negin, Martiniuk, & Jan, 2017; Ciccone, Vian, Maurer, & Bradley, 2014; Emerson, 2018; Glandon, Meghani, Jessani, Qiu, & Bennett, 2018; Siddiqi et al., 2009; Swanson et al., 2015; Tangcharoensathien, Srisookwatana, Pinprateep, Posayanonda, & Patcharanarumol, 2017).

The challenge of collaboration becomes more acute in the context of authoritarian or semi-authoritarian regimes which do not possess a culture of participatory policy making. In these settings, cultural barriers coupled with structural barriers adversely contribute toward a policy environment which is not conducive to the formation and persistence of policy networks. In recent years, especially since 2015, Turkey has been classified as an "open electorally competitive authoritarian regime" (Howlett & Tosun, 2018) or simply a "competitive authoritarian regime" (Esen & Gümüşçü, 2016, 2018). In this context, statism is perceived as the dominant pattern of policy making approach (Bölükbaşı & Ertuğal, 2018). In Turkey, "[h]istorically, state actors have displayed deep-seated distrust towards societal interests" (Bölükbaşı & Ertuğal, 2018, p. 11), and, as a result, policy making is largely closed to the participation of societal actors with some minimal exceptions at the policy implementation stage. Clearly, scholars should not dismiss the accounts on "the statist policy style" (Bölükbaşı & Ertuğal, 2018) or the purported "Napoleonic administrative tradition" (Turc, Guenoun, Rodrigues, Demirkaya, & Dupuis, 2016) which highlight the structural and cultural factors (e.g., system level factors) that influence politics and policy making in Turkey.

Within this framework, the aim of this chapter is to offer a spectrum of cross-sectoral arrangements that take place within the Turkish health sector by focusing on those arrangements that fail to become collaborative as defined in this study. These cross-sectoral arrangements are often misconceived as practices of collaborative policy making or policy networks particularly among policy practitioners. Scholarly research, on the other hand, has been more critical toward these arrangements, primarily due to the scepticism about the nature and effectiveness of the societal actors' involvement in policy processes. Previous research has described NGO involvement in policy making in Turkey as cases of "participation on paper" or cases of participation only in appearance and discourse without any genuine impact on policy processes (Paker, Adaman, Kadirbeyoğlu, & Özkaynak, 2013, p. 76). Field research conducted for the purpose of this examination reveals three types of cross-sectoral arrangements within the health sector which will be referred to as *consultative networks, cluster networks, patronage networks* (see Fig. 2) in this study. While a significant portion of scholarly attention has investigated patronage or clientelist networks as long-standing patterns in Turkish politics, less attention has been given to consultative and cluster networks as relatively new instruments of policy making pronounced particularly after the AKP rise to power. The rest of the chapter is organized as follows. The first, second, and third sections provide a spectrum of cross-sectoral arrangements within the health sector since 2003 in Turkey by investigating three practices that fall short of becoming collaborative based on the field research conducted for the purpose of this study. The final concluding section evaluates the findings presented in the previous sections and discusses the inherited structural and cultural barriers that impede network collaboration in Turkey.

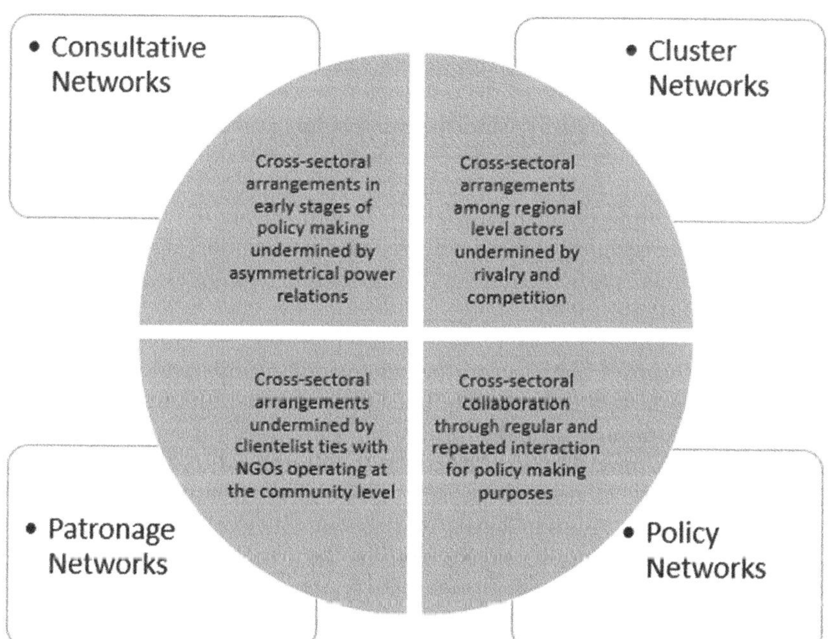

Fig. 2. Cross-Sectoral Arrangements within the Turkish Health Sector.

Consultative Networks: Policy Collaboration or Policy Legitimation?

Much has been said about the function of consultations during the stage of policy formulation and implementation at the national, local, and supranational levels of governance such as the case of European Commission open consultations (Van Ballaert, 2017). Despite their prominence, open and broad-scale public consultations are beyond the scope of this study which focuses on external stakeholder consultations with professional associations, business associations, research organizations, professional experts, or specialized NGOs, particularly at the stage of policy formulation. Generally, the extent to which governments undertake consultations with external stakeholders and the extent to which those consultations are used and translated into actionable policies depends upon multiple factors including the "complexity, newness, and salience of a proposal" (Van Ballaert, 2017) and the policy making styles of the countries under investigation (Toke & Nielsen, 2015) which returns scholarship to examine the issue of political and administrative culture. However, such findings do not have a conclusive nature. Governments in countries with a pluralistic policy tradition periodically choose to set aside consultations or arrange them for simply perfunctory purposes without a genuine intention to utilize them. For example, in the UK during the administration of Prime Minister Thatcher "there was consultation, but after the main policy decisions had been taken and on the government's terms" (Richardson, 2012, p. 316).

This study focuses on consultative processes carried out at the stage of health policy formulation in Turkey. Recent research entertains the idea of change in the public administration system toward more inclusive and transparent forms of governance, particularly due to the influence EU accession process (Bölükbaşı, Ertuğal, & Özçürümez, 2018). Nevertheless, scholars point out that "Turkey still has problems of participation in governance processes, both from outside (civil society) and inside (members of bureaucracy)" (Üstüner & Yavuz, 2018, p. 829) with regard to both to policy formulation and implementation processes. Policy formulation processes are notably dominated by the traditional statist policy style, and words such as "participation" or "consultation" remain an empty rhetoric (Bölükbaşı & Ertuğal, 2018):

> Typically government actors formulate policies unilaterally when drafting process is largely not open for participation of societal actors. Although formal consultation is provided for once legislative acts have been drafted, there is still no legal requirement on the part of the government for holding structured stakeholder consultation in legislative processes. The extent to which governments consult stakeholders is, thus, highly uneven and informal. (Bölükbaşı & Ertuğal, 2018, p. 12)

However, the research presented to date does not provide detailed accounts of specific procedures and instruments used in consultative processes at the stage of policy formulation. Considering this gap in the literature, this study aims at disentangling the intricacies of the consultative process at the stage of policy formulation. Field research reveals that policy consultation is manifested through multi-stakeholder meetings, roundtable workshop series and forums, special committees, or more specialized Health Technology Assessment (HTA) groups. Regarding the profile of societal actors attending consultative processes, field research reveals that only a limited number of professional associations or specialized NGOs are included in policy consultations. First, only a few professional associations within the health sector have the necessary expertise and know how needed to contribute to policy making at the national level, implying the lack of NGO input to policy formulation processes. Secondly, lack of willingness to contribute to policy making is another equally problematic issue. The majority of NGOs are project-based, service-oriented organizations that compete for funding against each other with no intention to be involved in policy making processes. Third, professional associations are completely excluded or included on a selective basis. Some professional associations reveal that they are not incorporated into the early stages of policy formulation, and, consequently, do not contribute to decision-making. Other professional associations are invited by the central government to attend multi-stakeholder consultative meetings in order to discuss already formulated policy proposals which will be discussed below.

This study focuses on two types of consultative networks within the Turkish health sector established in the policy sub-areas of pharmaceutical and medical device industry which this study argues best illustrate the nature of policy consultations within the Turkish health sector. These consultative networks take the form (a) broad multi-stakeholder meetings and (b) specialized committees that deal with specific policy issues in the policy sub-areas of pharmaceutical and medical device industry. The function of these networks is to serve as venues of policy consultation among central government, professional associations, private sector representatives (e.g., small and medium size enterprises/SMEs) and research institutions, and eventually, to enhance performance and productivity in the sectors of pharmaceuticals and medical devices.

At the outset, *broad multi-stakeholder meetings* organized by the Turkish Medicines and Medical Devices Agency (TMMDA) host representatives from the pharmaceutical industry and medical devices industry in two separate settings. The objective of these meetings is to boost communication between state and non-state actors and collectively tackle some of the problems and challenges within the respective policy sectors. These encounters take the form of policy roundtable meetings or cross-sectoral dialogue hubs. Despite their prominence, these platforms are loosely organized, and they generate no translatable outcomes into policy proposals. Attending professional associations are not fully informed about the purpose of the meetings. As a result, they are often unprepared or have only vague recommendations that are not translated into concrete policies. Therefore, these meetings serve the purpose of opinion exchange rather than expertise exchange and end up as ad hoc, sporadic, and decorative cross-sectoral arrangements that camouflage hierarchical and centralized forms of policy making. Considering their demonstrative and perfunctory nature, these networks will be referred to as *empty networks* in this study. Despite efforts to incorporate non-governmental actors, the central government has the final say on policy formulation. Moreover, broad multi-stakeholder meetings carry the risk of turning into venues that engender tension, conflict, and distrust. During one of the meetings attended by the researcher (2015),[1] the private sector representatives openly questioned the role of the meetings for serving no practical purposes and lacking any impact on policy making processes. Toward the end, the meeting took the form of conflictual confrontation among some of the participants, leaving no room for consensual problem solving.

Specialized committees were established initially by the former Ministry of Development[2] in the form of cross-sectoral arrangements within the policy sub-area of medical industry.[3] Subsequently, the central government in Turkey was very receptive in adapting the method of HTA which is a relatively novel instrument that evaluates new technologies used in healthcare services. HTA "primarily targets to guide policy making, in reality, it aims to inform all of the parties related to the health technology in question" (Ministry of Health, 2013). HTA is utilized by committees specialized in technology assessment,[4] established by the Ministry of Health since 2013 with the formation of the Health Technology Assessment Department under the General Directorate of Health Research. Scholarly research is supportive of HTA as a policy instrument. However, there are doubts about their policy effectiveness. Recent research notes that "HTA is expected to play a role guiding policy makers to increase the value of investments" (Kahveci, Koç, & Küçük, 2017, p. 407) and invites health policy makers to "utilize health technology assessment in their … decision-making processes" (Yilmaz, Koç, Çil, & Kahveci, 2017, p. 21). Both these statements imply that HTA is a constructive yet underestimated instrument in terms of its potential to affect policy making. Specialized committees have an essentially innovative nature encouraging stakeholder participation in policy making. Their focus is often concentrated on one single policy issue, and they strategically contribute to evidence-based health policy making. Yet, in practice, they turn out to be incredibly selective in terms of actors being involved and not very effective in providing practical policy recommendations and future directions for upcoming policies. Previous research has shown that

---

[1]The researcher attended the meeting as an observer invited the head of the TMMDA for research purposes.

[2]The Ministry of Development was founded in 2011 and was closed in 2018 after the institutional changes of the executive presidential system came into effect.

[3]http://www.seis.org.tr/docs/daha-cok-uretmeliyiz/kalkinma-plani/tibbi-cihaz-ve-tibbi-malzeme-calisma-grubu-raporu.pdf; file:///C:/Users/Julinda/Documents/PhD%20Dissertation/Dissertation/Field%20Research/Health%20subpolicy%20areas%20Problem%20Driven%20Networks%20emerge%20under%20complex%20circumstances/Politika%20hazirlama%20gelistirme%20innovation%20ulusal%20aglari/%C4%B0la%C3%A7%20%C3%87al%C4%B1%C5%9Fma%20Grubu%20Raporu.pdf

[4]Technology Assessment Department, General Directorate of Health Research, MoH, Topic Selection Commission/HTA Consulting Commission: http://www.hta.gov.tr/EN/Default.aspx.

continuous consultation with a limited number of societal actors might negatively influence overall policy effectiveness. "[L]imited community group resources and too many consultative exercises can lead to diminishing return and ineffectiveness if they are utilized too often" (Howlett, 2011, p. 158). In addition to effectiveness issues, government consultations with a select number of actors have another limitation. These consultative networks risk becoming politicized venues where only a selected group of professional associations that do not oppose the government policies are invited in order to legitimize already designed policies.

Overall, the aforementioned consultative networks disguise centralized, hierarchical, and asymmetrical forms of policy making, and as a result, do not qualify as forms of network collaboration as defined by this study. On paper, consultative networks are multi-stakeholder platforms established to enhance evidence-based health policy making through scientific and technical knowledge sharing; however, in practice, they serve the purpose of legitimation of already designed policies. Consultative networks occur primarily behind closed doors and have no measurable impact on policy making processes and/or outcomes. Besides transparency and accountability issues, the field research shows that consultative networks have minimum or no bottom-up input to policy making. To summarize, policy formulation either takes place through a fast-paced process within the state apparatus or involves consultation with societal actors which is open to debate concerning issues of transparency, accountability, and effectiveness.

Government hesitation against institutionalized and consensus-oriented consultations with impact on policy making may be due to government's sceptical attitude toward non-state actors, due to the aspiration to preserve the legacy of statist tradition in health policy making or the lack of political willingness to engage in lengthy and costly cross-sectoral arrangements manifested in the form of bureaucratic inertia. Regardless of the motivation, consultative networks investigated in this study do not qualify as cases of network collaboration. Despite lacking a genuine collaborative dynamic, multi-stakeholder meetings and specialized committees should not be seen in a completely negative light. Given that these arrangements serve as venues that promote deliberation at the cross-sectoral level, they have the potential to turn into networks with impact on policy making if they become truly representative and involve mechanisms of common decision-making among stakeholders.

Cluster Networks: Policy Collaboration or Deepening Fragmentation?

Clusters have been defined as "geographic concentrations of interconnected companies and institutions in a particular field, linked by commonalities and complementarities" (Porter, 1998, p. 78). Such geographic concentrations must provide "active channels for business transactions, dialogue, and communications" (Rosenfeld, 1997, p. 10) which serve as the meeting point between cluster and network approaches that seem to be two closely intertwined concepts. Considering the similarities between the two, cluster and network analysis have been used concurrently in previous research (Timur & Getz, 2008). Similar to policy networks clusters facilitate cross-sectoral collaboration of primarily geographically proximate actors. Within the Turkish health sector, clusters have been established mainly in the policy sub-areas of (a) health tourism and (b) the medical industry. These clusters have led to the development of broad networks of actors composed of provincial and sub-provincial organizations; however, their impact on policy making processes is questionable.

The development of clusters at the regional level has expanded in parallel with the development of regional development agencies (RDAs).[5] The latter "bring together local public and private actors including governors, mayors, chambers of industry and commerce and non-governmental organizations representing the private sector and/or civil society" (Bölükbaşı & Ertuğal, 2018, p. 9), with the purpose of "regional development planning and implementation by using public resources" (Bölükbaşı & Ertuğal, 2018, p. 9). RDAs are structurally linked to the central government. Nevertheless, they are expected operate independently at the regional level which contributes to their semi-public or hybrid status. RDAs are considered to play a leading role in cluster development projects in Turkey (Bulu & Yalçıntaş, 2015, p. 337). Both clusters and RDAs aim at increasing the competitive advantage of the region focusing on certain priority development areas and encouraging network collaboration among various actors at the regional level through repeated thematic workshops and round table meetings. In this way, both clusters and RDAs are expected to contribute to the formation of a *regional policy space* in the policy sub-areas of health tourism and medical industry.

Initially, cluster meetings in the field of health tourism in Turkey are organized with representatives of the central government at the local level, RDA representatives, university researchers, private sector representatives, and NGOs. Interviews indicate that health tourism clusters are in principle important platforms that facilitate multi-stakeholder engagement at the regional level. However, they reveal that these platforms have practically failed to meet their initial objectives. Considering different stages of cluster formation and development, health tourism clusters with headquarters in Antalya, Izmir, and Adana have not progressed beyond the initial stage of goal setting and have not became collaborative in the true sense of the word. Against this background, the main line of criticism is directed toward central government representatives at the local level (i.e., public actors) and RDAs (i.e., semi-public actors) for carrying the main responsibility, and yet, not playing a constructive role in organizing collaborative efforts among stakeholders at the regional level.

The involvement of the public actors at the local level has been a source of criticism repeated several times during the interviews. According to the interviewees, the government's hands off approach leads to mobilization and coordination problems among actors in the region. For instance, the local health authority,

---

[5]Kalkınma Ajanslarının Kuruluşu, Koordinasyonu ve Görevleri Hakkında Kanun (Law on the Establishment, Coordination and Tasks of Development Agencies), No. 26074, 8 February 2006: http://www.resmigazete.gov.tr/eskiler/2006/02/20060208-1.htm.

namely the Provincial Directorate of Health (İl Sağlık Müdürlüğü), has been criticized for failing to encourage cluster collaboration within the health tourism sector. During the interviews, RDA representatives call for more central governmental involvement in cluster activities emphasizing the critical role of public actors in coordinating regional (i.e., provincial and sub-provincial) level actors. In one of the interviews the governor is perceived as the "elder brother," who has the necessary qualities to keep the balance among all the stakeholders and, therefore, the only legitimate and capable actor to be given leadership roles. These statements imply that, in spite of all effort to create a local policy space, local level actors (i.e., semi-public, private, and voluntary) look upon the central government for guidance and leadership. Interviews indicate that private sector representatives do not have leadership roles within health tourism clusters, and, on top of it, they lack the motivation and overall commitment to collaborate due to ongoing business competition and rivalries in the region. As a result, cluster meetings focus on the specific concerns and demands of the private sector representatives, thus overshadowing issues of common interest regarding overall regional competitiveness.

RDAs have also been a target of criticism. Theoretically, RDAs serve as a bridge between national policy priorities set by the central government and regional/local interests. RDAs must address the needs of the locally owned SMEs and encourage network collaboration at the regional level. Operating in 26 regions in Turkey, RDAs are expected to "analyze their regions and support projects in order to create a more competitive economic environment" (Bulu & Yalçıntaş, 2015, p. 334). Despite their prominence, field research shows that RDAs play an ambiguous role within the framework of regional, health tourism development. Interviews indicate that RDAs do not play a particularly active role in encouraging actor collaboration at the regional level and supporting health tourism clusters. Moreover, their degree of autonomy from the central government is questionable. Instead of minimizing the role of the central government in the region, these agencies seem to promote it further with "the public actors, especially the governors, [being] at the forefront of decision-making processes" (Bölükbaşı & Ertuğal, 2018, p. 9).

Informed by the debates in the literature, health tourism clusters in Turkey do not go beyond the first stage of collaboration where "the key direction of innovative policy" (Mindlin, Zhukov, Prokhorova, Shutilov, & Belova, 2016, p. 264) is formed. Despite their initial expectations, regional health tourism clusters have engendered a series of counterproductive meetings with no concrete policy outcomes. Interviews indicate that the actors attending cluster meetings are not clear about the *raison d'être* of this type of multi-stakeholder interaction. Extrapolated from the literature, health tourism clusters in Turkey can be categorized under potential or would-be clusters where members "lack too many attributes to achieve the advantages of clusters" (Rosenfeld, 1997, p. 12). In some cases, clusters could not be maintained in the long run due to competing channels of authority, role confusion, lack of a shared vision, lack of commitment, lack of coordination, lack of political support, and on-going rivalries among cluster members. Over time, interaction within these clusters stopped for being ineffective and, to some extent, conflict driven.

Overall, health tourism clusters operate over a fragmented terrain that is not conducive to cross-sectoral network collaboration. Interviews suggest that one way to overcome collective action problems within clusters is to design a common strategy of regional health tourism development which will eventually increase the individual benefits of all cluster members. A common policy of regional health tourism would facilitate collaboration among actors who would consider themselves as partners rather than rivals. Another interviewee argued that the cluster meetings would turn into effective venues of collaboration only if they sparked interest among participants from the start, especially by giving concrete examples of successful collaborative projects and practices abroad. Previous successful cases would serve as an incentive to work together toward common goals in a synergetic fashion. Otherwise, private sector actors would feel alienated from the whole process which actually happened in the cases under consideration. Despite initial expectations, cluster meetings led to further fragmentation in the health tourism sector by making the idea of collaboration at the regional level less appealing to cluster members.

Another type of cluster interaction takes place within the sector of medical industry. Medical industry clusters are channels where SMEs can voice their grievances, address common problems, and tackle sector related challenges. In addition, medical clusters intend to spur product innovation and create a knowledge based industry through constant interaction with research institutions, particularly universities. Finally, medical industry clusters can be perceived as an instrument of cost control by the government by promoting corporate social responsibility among firms in the medical industrial sector. Therefore, medical industry clusters serve as venues where interests of businesses, universities, and governments conspicuously converge through the well-known triple helix model of development, witnessed in many developed countries, especially the United States (Etzkowitz & Zhou, 2017). In theory, the advantage of medical industry clusters is that they bring government and university representatives together with private firms, particularly SMEs operating in the medical industry sector and establish linkages between them through various channels of communication and dialogue including face-to-face contact made possible by geographical proximity at the regional level. Field research shows that medical industry clusters in Turkey have been formed in some pioneering cities such as Istanbul, Ankara, and Samsun.[6]

The interviews reveal that the relation between the central government and the cluster members is particularly tension driven. Cluster members consider the governmental approach toward SMEs as unsupportive or, at best, hesitant toward cooperation. They insist that the government should redirect the attention toward SMEs and institutionalize the collaboration with the industrial clusters in order to contribute the economic development of Turkey. The relations between cluster members and the university representatives seem to be

[6]Most of the findings in the section of medical industry clusters are based on the field research of OSTIM Medical Industry Cluster based in Ankara.

more cooperative. Periodically, medical clusters engage in common research and development projects with university researchers. Nevertheless, besides such sporadic encounters active channels of communication through network collaboration with impact on policy processes are largely missing. High level bureaucrats working in the public sector, on the other hand, argue that they are willing to support SMEs through offset applications. However, these companies do not fulfill the basic criteria of healthcare production. They lack the necessary expertise, competence, know-how, and spirit of technological innovation, and ultimately, they are not competitive in the global markets. Moreover, these companies are constantly competing for government funds without due consideration to follow the guidelines and directives of the government in a cooperative fashion. Clearly, central government and private sector representatives do not recognize each other as legitimate partners that render collaborative efforts within medical industry clusters largely unproductive. All in all, interviews reveal that there is lack of mutual trust among all parties which negatively influences cluster interaction. Similar findings have been reported in an investigation of the medical industry cluster in Samsun, and according to these findings, the lack of trust and a lack of collaborative culture are serious challenges to cluster level innovation (Çetin, Tekmen, Karaahmetoğlu, & Torun, 2016).

To sum up, both health tourism and medical industry clusters have not achieved the anticipated effects in terms of actor mobilization, cross-sectoral collaboration, and policy action at the regional level. Not only do health tourism and medical industry clusters fall short of generating a network type of collaboration at the cross-sectoral level, but they also fall short of addressing the problems private firms have in their respective industries at the regional level. Whether this situation reflects the inability of the societal actors to build a common culture of entrepreneurial innovation and collaboration or the lack of active support from the public sector actors is open to debate. One thing is certain – the regional policy space in the policy sub-areas of health tourism and medical industry has not yet been formed in Turkey. This finding sits well with previous research which argues that the regional development plans, in general, "have largely failed to mobilise regional partnerships among the public, private, and civil society actors, while the amount of financial resources distributed are completely inadequate to address developmental needs" (Bölükbaşı et al., 2018, p. 151).

Patronage Networks: Policy Collaboration or Political Expediency?

This section investigates patronage networks formed within the policy sub-area of community-based health and social services in Turkey. Before discussing patronage networks, an examination is provided about community-based health and social services including policy sub-areas conducive to network formation. Due to trends such as aging population and rising hospital service costs, community-based health and social services have become one of the most prominent issues within the field of health in the recent years. Being substantial in terms of number stakeholders, multitude of problems, and variety of implementable projects, community-based health, and social services have turned into a fertile ground for the study of policy networks (Chaskin, 2001; Freudenberg et al., 1994; Isett & Provan, 2005; Keast, Mandell, Brown, & Woolcock, 2004; Mandell, 1999; Provan, Isett, & Milward, 2004; Provan & Milward, 995; Roussos & Fawcett, 2000). The majority of these studies investigate health care and social services in the US cities, with a particular focus on community mental health networks. In such cases, public, private, and voluntary local level actors take advantage of community linkages and social sources of knowledge to build action networks at the neighborhood level.

Similar to other countries, the need for community-based health and social services has increased in Turkey. Since 2004, the amount of funds allocated for social services at the local level has increased significantly through hybrid bodies such as Social Assistance and Solidarity Foundations (SYDVs). Following the establishment of the Ministry of Family and Social Policies in 2011 (MoFSP), new departments responsible for community level social services such as the Directorate General for Child Services, the Directorate General for Persons with Disabilities and Elderly Services, and the Directorate General for Family and Community Services were established. The first legal arrangement on community health services was the "Regulation on the Delivery of Home Care Services" issued by the Ministry of Health in 2005.[7] This regulation transferred the right for service delivery in the area of home care to private healthcare providers. A great deal of community-based health and social services has been carried out under the umbrella of Social Services and Child Protection Agency (SHÇEK). Some services associated with SHÇEK have been provided through voluntary contributions or through *cooperation protocols* signed with public agencies and organizations, universities, and non-governmental organizations. Another important initiative has been the establishment of Community Mental Health Centers (CMHCs), active in Turkey since 2011,[8] which are encouraged to engage in collaboration with other actors at the local level including other health service providers, municipalities, NGOs, and research institutes. Even though the central government has to some extent withdrawn from service delivery at the local level, the central government has a crucial role in the design, initiation, and funding of projects on community-based health services. Despite recent developments, local government, NGO, and private sector involvement in community healthcare services is still low in Turkey. In most of the cases, the involvement of municipalities, non-governmental, and non-profit actors is confined to management of rehabilitation centers, homecare, and childcare services.

During the field research, interviewees call for mote NGO involvement in the provision of health and social services at the community level. NGOs are

---

[7]Evde Bakim Hizmetleri Sunumu Hakkinda Yönetmelik, Resmî Gazete Tarihi: 10.03.2005 Resmî Gazete Sayısı: 25751: http://www.mevzuat.gov.tr/Metin.Aspx?MevzuatKod=7.5.7542&MevzuatIliski=0&sourceXmlSearch=evde%20bak%C4%B1m.

[8]TC. Sağlık Bakanlığı. Toplum Ruh Sağlığı Merkezleri Hakkında Yönerge, 2011; https://www.saglik.gov.tr/TR,11269/toplum-ruh-sagligi-merkezleri-hakkinda-yonerge.html

perceived as an irreplaceable source of information because they can best assess individual level needs and provide critical information about local communities. They are also best equipped to provide community-based services by focusing on the specific needs and experiences of the individuals (i.e., the elderly, the poor, and children). Service oriented non-governmental organizations are expected to serve as a bridge between the government and the society within the framework of community-based health and social services. Contrary to this expectation, the field research demonstrates that the influence of non-state actors on policy making processes is marginal if not absent within this policy sub-area. Field research reveals that cross-sectoral interaction at the community level is dominated by informal connections between the government and a handful of NGOs which take the form of patronage networks. The selected voluntary organizations have privileged access to funding on community-based projects in return for political support and loyalty.

Within this framework, this study investigates the Collaborative Project on In-Home Health Care Services (Evde Sağlık ve Bakım İşbirliği Projesi) which serves as an example to illustrate the dynamics within local patronage networks. This project which has been designed at the national level and applied at the community level consists of multiple local level platforms located in geographically dispersed regions of Turkey. The first pilot project was launched in the province of Bolu through an implementation plan anticipated to be transferred to other cities in Turkey. The actors involved in this collaborative project at the local level are the Governorship of Bolu (Bolu Valiliği), the Bolu Municapality (Bolu Belediye Başkanlığı), the Provincial Health Directorate (İl Sağlık Müdürlüğü), Social Assistance and Solidarity Foundation running under the Bolu Governorship (Bolu İli Sosyal Yardımlaşma ve Dayanışma Vakfı, SYDV), Provincial Directorate of Health and Social Policies (Aile ve Sosyal Politikalar İl Müdürlüğü), Provincial Directorate of the Turkish Red Crescent (Türk Kızılayı Bolu Şube Başkanlığı), and a few societal actors including Home Health Care and Social Services Organization (Evde Sağlık ve Sosyal Hizmetler Derneği/EVSAD). This project is expected to increase the effectiveness of community-based health and social services through collaboration within a horizontal network structure at the local level, particularly through the close cooperation of public actors and NGOs.

Despite initial aspirations, the interaction among actors has not turned into genuine network collaboration with policy impact at the local level. In this case, interaction takes place within a clientelist web of relations where informal, interpersonal relations prevail upon formal channels of communication. Civil society organizations involved in this cross-sectoral collaboration are selected by the central government on the basis of allegiance to the ruling party and serve their political agenda by offering health and social services at the local level. The role of the central government and local government representatives within this network is to legitimize the essentially clientelist relationship by financing such projects through state funds. The role of involved NGOs in the project is to serve as extended party channels to reach citizens through selective services. The NGOs closely aligned with the government will be referred to as *ancillary organizations* here. The role of these ancillary organizations, specialized in service provision at the community level, is to ensure that the ruling party preserves its legitimacy and popularity within its constituency rather than contribute to bottom-up approach in the delivery of in-home healthcare services. Previous research has shown that "overly close alignment of such groups [civil society groups] with government is likely to undermine their legitimacy and limit their ability to press for social change" – a situation often encountered in low- and middle-income countries (Rasanathan, Atkins, Mwansambo, Soucat, & Bennett, 2018, p. 3).

Of great importance is the role of particular individuals working in the aforementioned ancillary organizations. Members of these organizations, who have worked or are still working in public offices (e.g., overlapping memberships), have the necessary connections with government officials, and possess the expertise to manage the projects at hand. These individuals play a significant role as mediators who go beyond organizational boundaries and serve as contact points between public and voluntary organizations. These individuals have been previously recognized in the literature as "boundary role persons" or "individuals who provide the linking mechanism across organizational boundaries" (Currall & Judge, 1995, p. 152). Besides serving as bridges across organizations, these individuals contribute toward the legitimation of the NGOs they represent, particularly in settings where public actors are largely sceptical of NGO involvement in policy making processes. Subsequently, NGOs involved in collaborative projects serve as extended channels of the ruling party rather than autonomous entities that contribute to policy making through bottom-up impulse. Given this context, scholars may discuss the presence of a clientelist structure that achieves the short-term interests of the involved actors, particularly the ruling political party.

Based on the findings above, patronage networks do not involve formal inter-organizational platforms of communication and common decision-making, but rather informal inter-personal linkages between mainly governmental and non-governmental organizations linked with the ruling party. Linkages within patronage networks are built and maintained by particular individuals who serve as contact points between these organizations. These findings conform well with previous research which argues that co-optation is maintained at the sub-national level of governance in Turkey through "extensive local networks among local branches of the ruling party, municipalities, local businesses and non-governmental organizations which are linked to the government and with often overlapping memberships" (Bölükbaşı & Ertuğal, 2018, p. 12). Considering the above, it would be misleading to talk about policy networks or even a formal structure of multi-stakeholder cooperation within the policy sub-area of community-based health and social services in Turkey. The role of pro-government, service-oriented NGOs at the community level is too political to have any policy impact. In brief, patronage networks in the area of community-based health and social services are another territory where the political expediency of the ruling party eclipses policy action based on the principles of universality, equity, and transparency.

The findings in the area of on in-home healthcare services are unsurprising considering that local level politics has for years been dominated by pork and barrel spending in Turkey. Patronage, clientelism, and political preferentialism represent long-standing phenomena in Turkish political and administrative culture which have been expanded after the AKP rise to power (Gürakar & Bircan, 2018; Sayari, 2014). The AKP maintained this tradition and even reinforced it by promulgating itself as a service oriented party that has been directly involved in the provision of social and health services by favoring selected segments of society at the community level in return for political support (Aytaç, 2014; Zencirci, 2015a, 2015b). These patterns have been observed the most in the relationship between public and voluntary actors which is marked by "prevalence of patronage networks [and] state scepticism toward and underestimation of civil society" (Özçetin & Özer, 2015, p. 16).

The root cause for the persistence of patronage networks at the local level goes back to the absence of a *local policy space* in Turkey which creates an opportunity for the undue and overly politicized interference of the central government in many policy areas, in this case, community-based health and social services. Hence, in practice, local projects are centrally orchestrated, and the involved organizations serve as institutional extensions of the central government and the ruling party. It is within this institutional framework in which patronage networks still prevail which contributes to the development of a system of partiality that distributes social benefits to specific groups in the society and, eventually, paves the way to the erosion of social policy at the local level. This problem may be resolved if local governments (i.e., municipalities) are vested with more legal authority and responsibilities in the field of health and social services through social policy decentralization. Some interviewees argue that municipalities should bear the primary responsibility in providing community-based health and social services following the example of developed countries. However, this is a challenging if not daunting task if one considers that local governments in Turkey are under the "over-exercised administrative tutelage of the center and their strict monitoring and control from above" (Üstüner & Yavuz, 2018, p. 829). In addition to current capacity limitations, municipalities lack the necessary vision, motivation, and willingness to supervise and monitor health and social service programs at the local level in an autonomous fashion. As mentioned in previous research on local governments in Turkey, "municipalities will struggle against cognitive barriers to acting independently" (Turc et al., 2016, p. 133).

As a final note, it should be emphasized that decentralization, through the empowerment of the local government, does not automatically lead to supplementary space for societal involvement and better quality in the provision of community-based health and social services. This is especially true if local governments are not "subjected to stricter audit and control mechanisms" which renders them "new sites of rent seeking and corruption controlled by the local elite" (Kadirbeyoğlu, 2017, p. 289). Local governments should incorporate incentive-based and bottom-up channels for volunteering which facilitate the collective action of public, private, and voluntary organizations, particularly neighborhood organizations, as well as local inhabitants. Research on community based health initiatives shows that the most effective type cooperation at the community level takes place when interaction among actors is integrated and systematically organized (Provan, Huang, & Milward, 2009; Provan & Milward, 1995), a situation that contributes significantly to the formation of community capacity (Chaskin, 2001).

Previous research suggests that community capacity building in the area of urban regeneration in Turkey is effective when coupled with a series of trainings for local government professionals and local community (Özçevik, Beygo, & Akçakaya, 2010). Further studies should be conducted to examine the nature and role of volunteering as well as community capacity on the effectiveness of community-based health and social services in Turkey.

Conclusion

Previous research points out that:

> the emergence of new forms of governance in local spaces may be exaggerated if all types of network arrangements are taken as evidence of a transformation from government to governance. (Parker, 2007, p.129)

Cross-sectoral arrangements can be confused with networked forms of governance due to the multitude of actors involved and issues tackled, and yet, a close examination of these arrangements reveals that they lack the mechanisms of collaboration discussed in the previous chapter. This chapter provides an overview of the cross-sectoral arrangements other than policy networks. Juxtaposition of all cross-sectoral arrangements has a twofold purpose. First, it enhances our understanding of policy networks as platforms of cross-sectoral collaboration with some measurable impact on policy making. Second, it contributes toward a better understanding of the underlying dynamics of relationships and processes that hinder policy collaboration within the Turkish health sector, including factors pertaining to the Turkish political and administrative culture such as patronage, clientelism, and opportunism, as well as, structural barriers such as on-going rivalries and fragmentation that hinder collaboration particularly at the regional level

Three types of networking that fail to become collaborative have been identified: consultative, cluster, and patronage networks. In the case of consultative networks, stakeholders continue to meet in platforms arranged by the central government for demonstrative purposes in order to legitimize already designed policies and action plans. While these platforms involve cross-sectoral interaction during the policy formulation stage, they have no real impact on policy making processes and/or outcomes. In this case, centralized patterns of policy making and asymmetrical power relations are reproduced behind the façade of cross-sectoral collaboration. Cluster networks are more strategically organized in terms of goals to be pursued at the regional level. However, in practice these networks suffer from fragmented and frequently conflict-driven interaction that interrupts and eventually terminates the collaborative efforts without any final outcomes. At this point, cluster members do not perceive each other as legitimate partners mostly due to lack of mutual recognition of expertise and accumulated mistrust. Lastly, another type of cross-sectoral encounter takes places at the local level, namely in the area of community-based health and social services, through the close working relationship of the government with a selected number of NGOs which are either semi-public organizations (quasi-NGOs) or pro-government organizations (NGOs dedicated to the ruling party). These encounters, based on patron-client relations, lead to pro-government ventures arranged for political rather than policy purposes. As a result, these networks are referred to as *patronage networks* in this study.

Overall, these cases point out structural and cultural factors that impede the development of cross-sectoral collaboration within the health sector. Based on the cases under investigation, lingering structural and cultural barriers remain detrimental to the development of cross-sectoral collaboration within the health sector in Turkey at the national, regional, and local level. These factors include (a) statist bureaucratic tradition through centralized, hierarchical, and asymmetrical forms of policy making; (b) lack of legal requirements on the side of the central government to hold multi-stakeholder consultations during the stages of policy formulation and implementation; (c) restricted access to policy consultations suffering from issues of transparency, accountability, and effectiveness; (d) limited resources directed toward cross-sectoral projects; (e) weak institutional infrastructure that facilitates coordination with internal and external stakeholders; (f) bureaucratic inertia to get involved in costly and lengthy cross-sectoral arrangements; (g) lack of common culture of entrepreneurial innovation and collaboration among private sector actors at the regional level; (h) lack of adequate political and financial support toward regional clusters in the areas of medical industry and health tourism; (i) ambiguous role of RDAs as lead semi-public actors falling short of effectively organizing collaborative efforts in the region; (j) sceptical government attitude toward a cooperative relationship with civil society organizations; (k) government alignment with a selected number of NGOs (quasi-NGOs or pro-government NGOs); (l) limited NGO capacity to contribute to policy making within the health sector; (m) limited local government capacity to supervise health-related projects at the community level; (n) limited channels of voluntary action in the area of community-based health and social services; and (o) politicized intervention of the government at the local level particularly through clientelist ties with service-oriented NGOs semi-public foundations.

On a final note, the negative impact of structural and cultural impediments mentioned above can be mitigated through constant efforts to improve health governance at the national, regional, and local levels. This goal can be accomplished through continuous commitment of all stakeholders toward cross-sectoral network collaboration as an effective instrument of policy making.

Chapter 6

Conclusion: Leveraging Networks to Achieve Policy Collaboration

Abstract

This study is an attempt to (a) introduce Turkey as a country case with statist policy tradition and authoritarian political culture, yet, a growing importance of cross-sectoral collaboration in various policy areas, as an opportunity to conduct network research beyond advanced democracies (Chapter 1); (b) develop an integrated framework for the study of policy networks across country cases and policy settings at the sub-national level through the utilization of Network Collaborative Capacity Index (Chapter 2); (c) trace the contextual conditions that led to the formation of policy networks within the health sector from 2011 to 2015 in Turkey (Chapter 3); (d) examine those mechanisms that maximize collaboration along the structural, relational, and institutional dimensions of networks (Chapter 4); and (d) assess the cultural and structural impediments that inhibit cross-sectoral arrangements from becoming collaborative and influencing policy processes and outcomes (Chapter 5). This concluding chapter focuses on the theoretical significance as well as the practical effectiveness of the policy networks under consideration in an attempt to link the local practice of network collaboration with more general theories of governance.

Keywords: Applied policy research; collaboration; future studies; neo-institutionalism; network resilience; policy networks

> Despite contrary sentiments and certain efforts to unwind the network spring, the emergence of networks in public management is not a passing fad. (O'Toole, 1997, p. 47)

Network Policy Making within the Turkish Health Sector: Becoming Collaborative, 113 125

doi:10.1108/978-1-83867-094-820201007

Going Back to the Start: From Paradigm Shifts to Policy Practices

Prior to presenting the final remarks, it is essential to remind the reader of the ongoing discussions on Turkish politics outlined in the introductory chapter of the book. Together with the pro-democratic policy reforms launched in the aftermath of 2003 in Turkey, scholars of Turkish politics started asking questions regarding whether the Turkish political landscape been reshaped. Immersed within an enthusiastic atmosphere, well-established scholars of Turkish politics entertained the idea that the ruling AK Party holds potential for normalizing democracy through a "new social order on democratic foundations" (Insel, 2003, p. 306) and an "explicit liberal and democratic discourse" (Hale & Özbudun, 2009, p. 11). However, particularly after 2014, scholars have raised questions concerning Turkey relapsing toward an authoritarian or semi-authoritarian political regime. Özbudun (2014) confirms the Turkey's drift toward competitive authoritarianism since 2014 which "can be described as a period in which the AKP government made a sustained and systematic effort to establish its control over the judiciary" (p. 53). The two types of questions mentioned above head toward diametrically opposite directions; however, they represent the same research agenda which focuses on possible paradigm shifts at the system level in Turkey through macro-level institutional analysis. These accounts generate accurate pictures of the recent political developments in Turkey. Yet, constantly focusing on paradigm shifts within the Turkish political regime is likely to delude the researcher and the readers alike by bringing them back either to age-old debate on authoritarian political culture or to accounts that overemphasize the inevitable consequences of neoliberalism in Turkey influenced by ongoing debates within the field of political economy.

In search of transformative change, scholars of Turkish politics often loom between two extreme positions that presume trends toward either liberalism or authoritarianism, or they get stuck with *hybrid* political regimes that render Turkey, as it is often the case, a unique country that precludes any form of comparative assessment. This book aims at redirecting scholarly attention from paradigm shifts at the system level to practical mechanisms at the policy level. Following this logic, this book does not argue for the transformation of the political regime toward either liberalism or for the restoration of authoritarianism in Turkish politics. Instead, it focuses on the adoption of network policy making both in terms of policy thinking and policy practice within the Turkish health sector. To this end, the research seeks to understand the processes of network formation and persistence over time. The underlying assumption here is that real change in policy making patterns happens gradually and incrementally from simple perception to concrete policy design. If one considers the whole spectrum of policy making practices, the evidence presented in this study suggests only a few cases of genuine network collaboration, thus making the shift toward permanent modes of network governance within the Turkish health sector highly unlikely. However, as stated above, the researcher is less preoccupied with grandiose paradigm shifts and more interested in practical policy mechanisms.

This research position stems from the approach that defines networks as policy instruments that influence policy processes and outcomes as pathways toward an ideal mode of network governance that substitutes cumbersome formalities of the bureaucracies or competitive pressures of the markets. As previously stated in the literature "...the dinosaur scenario, emphasizing ... an inevitable and irreversible paradigmatic shift toward market or network organization, is wrong or insufficient" (Olsen, 2005, p. 17–18). Following a similar logic, "...local policy networks are insufficient in themselves to assure network governing in all settings" (Damgaard, 2006, p. 673). According to these statements, it would be hasty to conclude about an overall reconfiguration in the modes of governing or a redefinition of state–society relations. From a comparative perspective, Turkey is far from being a representative case for network governance, and yet, it is a case where policy networks have entered the jargon and practice of policy making. Hence, it would be an exaggeration to talk about the transformative potential of the current practices of network policy making in Turkey while in some other European countries, scholars are discussing the implications of too much network collaboration due to extended forms of policy networks described as "network of networks" (Assens & Lemeur, 2016, p. 26).

Field research conducted for the purpose of this study reveals that network thinking has been growing rapidly within the health sector, particularly within the public administration, since the introduction of health policy reforms in 2003. However, it is cross-sectoral collaboration carried out in the period between 2011 and 2015 which makes networks relevant policy tools instead of mere rhetorical devices used casually or metaphorically by policy practitioners. Refraining from seeking ambitious system level transformations, this study presents modest findings produced by micro- and meso-level analysis of network policy making. While this book does not suggest that centralized and hierarchical decision-making structures within the government are being replaced with horizontal and networked forms of governance, it demonstrates that networks have become an integral part of the practice of policy making within the Turkish health sector. This conclusion compels scholars of Turkish politics to expand the policy realm with new issues, actors, instruments, and concepts, and also incorporates Turkey into general governance debates. Going beyond the confines of Turkish politics, the findings of this study contradict the recent arguments that call into question the utility of policy networks as analytical concepts that can be used to explain policy making processes. Policy networks observed in the Turkish case seem to echo Laurence J. O'Toole's (1997) statement about treating networks seriously in public administration and public policy research. Moreover, the presence of policy networks in a country case such as Turkey challenges researchers to study the network type of policy collaboration as a phenomenon transferable across policy settings rather than a pattern exclusive to advanced democracies. Overall, this book is helpful for scholars with a general interest in collaborative policy making and health governance, students who strive to understand the complex dynamics of Turkish politics and policy making, and policy practitioners who aspire to develop collaboration skills and attitudes in their daily cross-sectoral encounters.

Theoretical Significance and Practical Effectiveness of Networks: Lessons from the Turkish Case

Network Formation: Networks as Deliberate Government Choices

It is difficult to identify a single cause that led to the formation of policy networks within the Turkish health sector from 2011 to 2015 which corresponds to the finalization of the first round of HTP reforms. There are many contextual factors which in conjunction led to the formation of policy networks. Among them, the most defining factor was the governmental choice to engage in cross-sectoral collaboration with representatives from the private and voluntary sectors. The rationale behind investing in cross-sectoral arrangements can be explained by the governmental willingness to maintain the legitimacy of the already implemented reforms through developing linkages with non-governmental actors during a period characterized by policy stability. This led to the creation of new institutional arrangements with a semi-autonomous status and new platforms conducive policy collaboration particularly in network prone areas such as public health, health tourism, and the medical industry. Besides being inherently multi-disciplinary domains that involve a multiplicity of actors, issues, and sectors, these policy areas were also placed high in the political agenda of the time as salient policy issues. Overall, multi-faceted programs launched by the government in the health policy sub-areas mentioned above, institutional re-organization toward a more dispersed management of the health system, and the presence of a conducive political, economic, and social environment paved the way to more stakeholder contribution to health policy making through mechanisms of risk, expertise, and information sharing.

Findings about network formation have implications for issues of policy stability and change particularly for countries in the developing world. The analysis conducted here suggests that policy networks emerge during times of policy stability rather than policy change or serious restructuring of the health system. In the latter scenario governments are inclined to act unilaterally and in an abrupt fashion in order to isolate policy initiatives from possible constraints from the political, economic, and social environment that might hamper reform efforts or slow down the policy implementation process. Within such circumstances, policy networks are to varying degrees state led ventures formed by the central government during periods of political stability and policy legitimacy. The post-reform period witnessed relatively low levels of criticisms of the government policies and increased levels of satisfaction with health policy services which contributed to self-affirmation of the government. In this context, the government aimed at consolidating reforms achievements by developing alliances with organizational stakeholders and establishing channels of communication with societal actors. These efforts contributed to growing number of cross-sectoral arrangements, including networks with measurable impact upon policy making processes until the year 2015 which records the re-centralization of the health system as well as reduced efforts to engage in cross-sectoral dialogue due to securitization and politicization of policy issues. Overall, this study adds to the debates on comparative public policy by linking policy networks to issues such as policy stability and policy legitimacy as two critical background factors that facilitate the formation of policy networks between 2011 and 2015 in Turkey.

On a final note, the formation of networks informs us about the nature of policy networks themselves. Previous debates often assume that policy networks are inevitable occurrences resulting from growing bottom-up input to policy making. Within this framework, networks are perceived as bottom-up designs that develop in an autonomous, natural, and organic fashion with almost inevitable and irreversible consequences to policy making and governing patterns. Considering the Turkish context, policy networks are not unanticipated breakthroughs that result from the bottom-up involvement of non-state actors in policy making in the strictest sense. Networks in this instance do not constitute truly bottom-up mechanisms of policy making. Taking into account their inception, networks are policy instruments that reflect the government's deliberate choice to engage in cross-sectoral collaboration during times of policy stability and legitimacy.

Network Capacity: Network as Instruments of Policy Collaboration

This study acknowledges that networks have a structural or organizational aspect concerning the geometry of interactions or nature of interdependence. However, the argument put forward in this examination is that excessive attention to the structural dimension of networks can obscure their value or significance as rather flexible instruments that facilitate policy collaboration as a process. Following this argument, this study frequently uses the phrase "network policy making" which evokes an ongoing process rather than "policy networks" which denotes a fixed structure in network research. In this study, network collaboration refers to process that helps parties from different policy sectors achieve consensual or mutually acceptable results with an impact on policy making process and outcomes. This definition makes networking an essentially collaborative processes with the purpose of health policy making. Collaboration with measurable policy impact serves as a common denominator for networks as instruments of policy collaboration and a benchmark distinguishing networks from other cross-sectoral arrangements that fail to become collaborative. In this case, failed attempts of policy collaboration refer to consultative, cluster, and patronage networks. By bringing Network Collaborative Capacity (NCC) to the fore, this study aims to bridge the gap between network debates and the broader literature on policy collaboration, more specifically cross-sectoral collaboration. In other words, this book suggests situating network analysis within a broader framework of collaborative governance.

Following this approach, this study identifies three success stories of network collaboration within the Turkish health sector with each representing a distinct model of network policy making. In this analysis, the index of NCC becomes a useful tool to identify different levels and types of collaboration leading to different forms of policy impact. Existing varieties of network policy making hinders the construction of a monolithic model applicable across all policy networks within the Turkish health sector. Methodologically, policy networks are best captured by typologies that reflect variation in terms of network structure, intra-network relations, and network institutionalization. Typologies require a research design that accounts for sub-national and sub-sectoral variations that focus on micro–meso level linkages fostering cross-sectoral collaboration rather than monolithic models applicable across policy settings and country cases.

In concrete terms, this book suggests three types of network policy making associated different levels of structural, relational and institutional capacity to collaborate. The first type of network policy making, shows that networks can turn into vehicles that diffuse policy innovation through intensive expertise sharing between government officials and university researchers, especially in the area of public health policy development, where academic entrepreneurs contribute to public policy formation (i.e., ÇPSSGP case). Public policy innovation requires a robust network structure through high levels of structural capacity and strong intra-network ties through high levels of relational capacity. The second type of network policy making indicates that networks are useful tools that lower the risk of huge investment projects through contract based enforcement, especially in the policy area of healthcare investments where the government and businesses share financial, technical, and human resources (i.e., public–private partnership (PPP) case). In this case, networks should operate within a clear legal and institutional framework that contributes to network resilience at the policy implementation stage. Therefore, this type of network policy making scores high in terms of institutional capacity to collaborate. Finally, networks serve the purpose of organizational-knowledge-sharing among a broad range of actors, especially in the policy area of health tourism, through close NGO–government partnership at the pre-operational phase of policy making (i.e., SATURK case). This type of network policy making does not exhibit particularly high levels of structural, relational, and institutional capacity to collaborate. Yet, it represents a flexible policy space that facilitates actor coordination through average levels of overall NCC.

Based on these findings, network policy impact can be organized around the themes of (a) policy innovation through evidence-based policy making at the policy formulation stage; (b) effective project operation through contract enforcement that involve risk sharing at the policy implementation stage; and finally (c) actor coordination through organizational-knowledge-sharing at the inter-stage between policy formulation and policy implementation. Based on the above, existing policy networks serve as opportunities that should not be squandered and should be developed by further leveraging their impact on policy making. It should be clarified here that aforementioned network benefits are not automatic outcomes of network policy making. On the contrary, they are products of intense and constant collective efforts of the involved stakeholders, which can be maximized by further strengthening the structural, relational, and institutional capacities of networks. Networks that display low levels of collaborative capacity can in time turn from tools of policy innovation to tools of policy inertia utilized by certain communities to avoid policy change from channels of effective policy making to time-consuming, lengthy, and inefficient encounters that add to the complexity of issues without any concrete policy outcomes and from policy spaces that facilitate ideational exchange and actor coordination to unstable constellations of actors that might reverse to market and/or hierarchical forms of policy making or even disintegrate altogether. Under such circumstances, network comparative advantages can easily turn into disadvantages which make networks policy instruments with minimum or no impact on policy making processes and outcomes.

This study demonstrates that not all cross-sectoral platforms result in network collaboration as defined in this study. One has to delve further into the structure and nature of relations in order to separate empty networks (i.e., those cross-sectoral platforms which are only gathered for demonstrative purposes) from cases of genuine network collaboration. This is exactly like the presence of collaboration serves as a common denominator for all policy networks, and its absence reduces cross-sectoral platforms into empty ventures with no impact on policy making processes and outcomes at minimum. Cross-sectoral arrangements that fails to become collaborative can have a detrimental effect on policy processes and outcomes leading to further organizational fragmentation within the health sector (i.e., cluster networks), politicization of policy making processes (i.e., consultative networks), and even patronage in social and health service delivery (i.e., patronage networks). Therefore, researchers should focus their attention on those factors that enhance or collaborative capacity by investigating the structural, relational, and institutional dimensions of networks, or conversely, those factors that impede network collaboration all together.

Network Durability: Making Networks Resilient in Unpredictable Policy Environments

Previous studies have shown that network durability holds at least equal value to network formation. This book concurs with this position by adding that durability can best be expressed through the term network resilience which refers to network persistence despite frequent and often unpredictable changes in political, economic, and social environments, a situation that is more pronounced in country cases such as Turkey. This study shows that the main challenge to collaboration within the Turkish health sector is not the absence of policy networks. On the contrary, networks are increasingly being formed as useful instruments of policy making. The field research reveals a rising awareness in the direction of network collaboration among policy practitioners. The notable challenge here is the persistence or maintenance of network collaboration over time throughout all the stages of policy making from agenda building to policy evaluation. Network collaboration observed within the Turkish health sector is often interrupted and stalled due to shifting political priorities, changing policy agendas, or simply termination of financial resources. This situation is exacerbated by constantly changing political appointees occupying higher-level positions within the bureaucracy who possess limited training and expertise concerning cross-sectoral projects with external stakeholders in addition to the lack of institutional memory within the Turkish administration issues that were brought up repeatedly during expert interviews.

This study suggests that networks follow a three stage schema of institutional resilience (see Fig. 3). First, the *entrepreneurship stage* refers to breaking the bureaucratic cycle of policy making through network formation (e.g., building support from the media, political, and societal elites). At this stage, the presence of a policy discourse that triggers cross-sectoral collaboration on

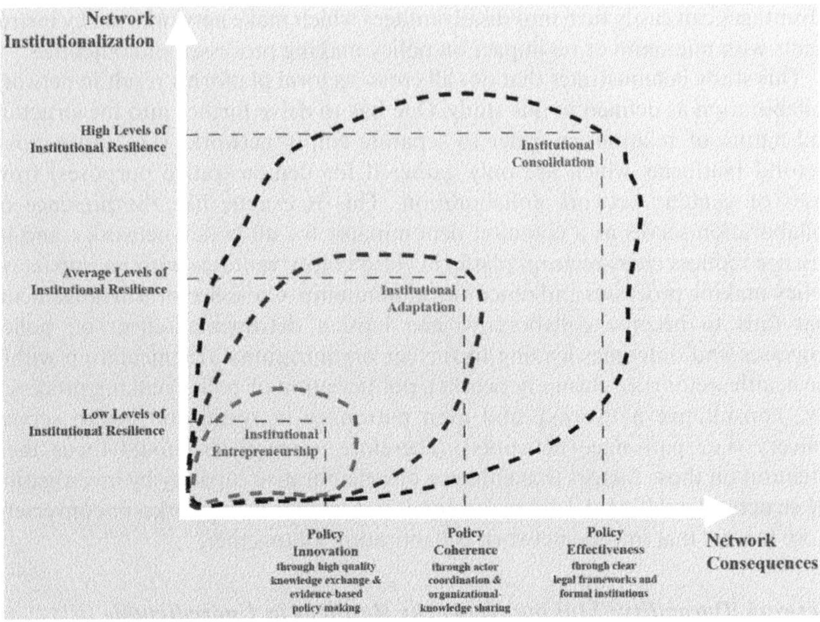

Fig. 3. Three Stages of Network Institutional Resilience.

the respective policy sub-area is adequate for network formation. In this study, this type of cross-sectoral collaboration leads to policy innovation through high quality knowledge-exchange among policy experts and professionals in early stages of policy making. Second, the *adaptation stage* refers to adjusting network dynamics to changing circumstances in the external political and economic environment (e.g., maintaining continuous support from prominent political leaders and state officials, business bases alliances, or political coalitions from the surrounding environment particularly between policy formulation and policy implementation). This is a challenging phase of network collaboration that requires careful management of both intra- and extra-network relations. As illustrated in this study, this type of cross-sectoral collaboration, when coupled with successful network management, enables actor coordination and organizational-knowledge-sharing, contributing to some degree of policy coherence between the stage of policy formulation and policy implementation. Third, the *consolidation stage* network refers to network persistence throughout the stages of policy making (e.g., network preservation through long-standing legal frameworks and formal institutions in the respective policy sub-area). At this stage of institutionalization, networks can turn into highly effective instruments of policy implementation. According to this approach, institutional resilience is very much contingent upon the embeddedness of the network in the external environment and constant efforts to receive external support from the media, societal elites, prominent political actors, high level officials, business-based alliances, and political coalitions until they are entrenched within relatively stable institutional and legal frameworks.

Following this logic, more advanced stages of network resilience are achieved when networks serve as channels that reflect already existing webs of actors and relationships such as business alliances and/or political collations in the broader economic and political environment and are backed by formal institutional structures. The example of PPPs best illustrates this argument. In spite of having weak internal ties, PPP based health construction projects are effective in terms of delivered policy outcomes as well as resilient in terms of network durability over time. Such networks, due to their capacity to serve as channels of interest mediation, can become more resilient over time and thrive in a constantly changing policy environment reaching the stage of institutional consolidation. On the contrary, despite having a robust internal structure concerning high levels of trust, common decision-making and connectedness at the network level Program for Improving Multi-Sectoral Health Responsibility (ÇPSSGP) has not generated a resilient institutional design to generate collaboration among stakeholders over time. As a result, this network has remained at the entrepreneurship stage with notably low levels of institutional resilience. SATURK, on the other hand, can be placed at the adaptation stage with average levels of institutional resilience.

Despite their prominence, exogenous factors central to neo-institutionalist approaches are often overlooked in network analysis which can take the form of snapshot analysis of the endogenous factors that affect policy networks. The argument put forward here is that the inward perspective into networks is not adequate to explain the lack of network persistence in the long run. Focusing on internal network structure makes perfect sense in those policy environments where network collaboration has already turned into a sustainable pattern of governance. However, this logic cannot be applied to those policy environments, such as the case of Turkey, where exogenous factors related to the broader institutional environment surrounding the network can influence not only intra-network relations but also the very persistence of collaboration over time. In this context, perspectives focusing solely on intra-network structure fall short of explaining why network instances do not turn into stable and long lasting patterns of collaborative governance. Overall, this study shows that the logic of network collaboration does not clash with the logic of institutional embeddedness in the broader, external environment advocated by the neo-institutional approaches. Therefore, the findings of this book concur with those studies that suggest the usefulness of incorporating neo-institutionalist approaches into network analysis, particularly in the context of constantly changing policy environments.[1]

Current Limitations and Future Directions

The Limits of Exploratory Network Analysis

Ritchie and Spencer (2002) identified four types of policy research using qualitative methods: "contextual," "diagnostic," "evaluative," and "strategic" (p. 174). The present study is primarily contextual and diagnostic and less evaluative and

---

[1]See Jens Blom-Hansen (1997) for the incorporation of new-institutionalism in the study of policy networks.

strategic in terms of research design as well as covered content. This was a deliberate choice made by the author when confronted with a lack of data and analysis specifically on policy networks and more generally cross-sectoral collaboration in the field public policy in Turkey. As a result, the present study offers policy implications; however, it is not a fully-fledged applied policy research which would require more extensive data sets as well as a wide range of methods including participant observations, surveys, and focus groups.

The content covered in this study provides a general overview of all types of cross-sectoral arrangements within the health sector, explores and examines the main dimensions of network collaboration, including the origins of network collaboration, the legal, and institutional framework upon which networks operate, the structure and nature of interaction within policy networks, the impact of network collaboration on policy, the main problems facing network participants, and identifies the factors that impede policy collaboration within cross-sectoral platforms. However, this study does not offer a detailed analysis concerning particular needs of each specific policy network or the specific action required to improve overall network performance. In addition, this study does not elaborate at length on issues such as network management, policy legitimacy, and democratic accountability. Strategic and evaluative research on individual policy programs should be carried out to shed light on these issue areas. Strategic and evaluative research design shifts the attention of research toward management related issues at different levels of the health system from health service delivery to health policy making, therefore, moving closer to applied policy research.

Furthermore, the findings presented in this study possess a limited potential for generalization at the national level of analysis. The comparability and reproducibility of the results obtained from semi-structured interviews can be difficult compared to other research methods such as surveys with closed-ended questions or more standardized research procedures. It should be noted here that the categories included in content analysis were measured by the researcher who engaged in analytical thinking throughout the coding process. The results obtained from this exercise which naturally involve some degree of interpretation have not yet been substantiated with data from follow up research. Considering these limitations, future studies might consider complementing interview data with focus group data which is a common practice in policy analysis. Focus group research with scholars would be productive in improving the quality of data and eventually refining the arguments presented in this study in order to achieve more conclusive results. First, focus group research would be helpful to discuss the responses of semi-structured interviews in line with scholarly judgment. Secondly, this type of research would offer insights on the particular role of universities and research institutes in health policy analysis in Turkey. A target group suitable for this type research would be one with university professors who are currently working in healthcare management programs and have experience in collaborative projects within the health sector (i.e., university–industry, university–government types of network collaboration).

Toward Strategic and Evaluative Network Analysis

Strategic research in network analysis can be carried out either through single case network analysis producing in-depth and systematic assessments tailored to offer specific policy recommendations or thematic studies focused on specific aspects of network collaboration, designed to overcome existing collaboration challenges. For example, future studies can focus on ongoing cases of policy collaboration such as SATURK in the policy sub-area of health tourism. The case of SATURK can serve as a laboratory to evaluate network management by examining the role of policy brokers in coordinating a wide range of actors at the pre-operational and implementation stages of policy making. Network management through policy brokers and information systems is a key aspect of network collaboration which was discussed yet it was not thoroughly elaborated in this study. Future studies should consider network management not only a catalyst that can maximize network collaboration but also a factor important to understand the role of policy networks as flexible and negotiable policy spaces.

Future research could evaluate the role of these policy brokers in synchronizing the shifting interests and policy agendas in the external environment with the dynamic reality inside policy networks. Policy brokers appear to have a critical role particularly in situations of network fatigue at the inter stage between policy formulation and policy implementation. During such times, policy brokers should address the needs and demands of network participants and at the same time accommodate the interests of stakeholders external to networks structure. Policy brokers have the advantage of connections with various stake holders within and outside the network structure are best suited to manage the network dynamics by maintaining or upholding the collaborative momentum and to reignite initial enthusiasm for collaboration. Future research should elaborate those management techniques such as communication strategies needed to facilitate information flow between organizations as well as coordination strategies needed to accommodate interests of different actors at all stages of policy making. One possible research avenue concerns information systems of communication utilized in existing network research.

Another possible area of research is the intersection of collaborative innovation[2] and policy networks. Here, researchers might focus their attention on those practices that facilitate collaborative innovation within networks particularly at the early stages of policy making. In this context, researchers can focus on those platforms that bridge the gap between "the so-called three cultures of research, policy, and practice" (Head, 2016, p. 478). Mitton, Adair, McKenzie, Patten, and Perry (2007) provide an comprehensive overview of the platforms that hold

---

[2]See the following published research on the topic of collaborative innovation. Agar and Sørensen (2018), Sørensen and Torfing (2016), Torfing (2019), and Torfing, Sørensen, and Røiseland (2019).

potential to turn into venues of knowledge transfer and exchange useful for evidence-based policy making in the area of health including:

> Face-to-face exchange (consultation, regular meetings) between decision makers and researchers/Education sessions for decision makers/Networks and communities of practice/Facilitated meetings between decision makers and researchers Interactive, multidisciplinary workshops/Interactive, multidisciplinary workshops/ Capacity building within health services and health delivery organizations/Web-based information, electronic communications/Steering committees (to integrate views of local experts into the design, conduct, and interpretation of research). (p. 744)

Future research should pay more attention to these platforms as potential venues for knowledge-exchange and transfer and evaluate the degree they facilitate collaborative innovation translatable to policy making. Within this research framework, special attention should be given to the issue of policy learning, in order to better understand the quality of interaction between researchers, policy makers, and policy practitioners.

Moreover, further attention should be given to the role of independent medical research institutes, health think tanks, and community-based service-oriented organizations in policy making processes. Based on the assumption that a cooperative process brings cooperative outcomes, increasing cross-sectoral collaboration with these non-governmental organizations would, in principle, contribute to the generation of consensus-based and legitimacy-oriented policy solutions in the area of health. However, the latter are very much dependent upon the development of a collaborative culture of policy making based upon continuous ideational exchange and shared learning with non-governmental organizations as well as pro-active involvement of these organizations to policy processes. To this end, researchers should focus their attention toward the role independent medical research institutes and health think tanks, through the study of similar examples set in developed countries where the organizations have a huge impact on strategic and evidence-based policy making (see Cairney & Oliver, 2017; Rycroft-Malone et al., 2016). Another research register should be developed on the development of community capacity in the area of healthcare services. This can be done through an assessment of local level actors including local NGOs, community leaders, and service providers with regard to their capacity to contribute to community-based health services through cross-sectoral collaborative projects (see Martsolf, Sloan, Villarruel, Mason, & Sullivan, 2018; Mattessich & Rausch, 2014).

Besides strategic type of research, evaluative research in network analysis can also contribute toward applied policy research in the area of health governance. Evaluative research can be conducted through a detailed assessment of network consequences based on criteria of policy effectiveness and political accountability. In the former case, network collaboration can be evaluated in terms of produced policy outcomes. The study of overall network effectiveness can be applied only in those network cases that have survived the stage of policy implementation.

Within this context, researchers can come up with frameworks for the evaluation of actual outcomes of cross-sectoral collaboration (see Provan & Milward, 2001). In this context, multi-sectoral policy evaluation and the way it affects future collaborative prospects in health policy may hold particular significance. Additionally, future studies can evaluate the degree to which networks carry the risk of engendering a contested domain of governance with no clear and sometimes overlapping chains of accountability and power distribution. Too many levels of interaction may shadow the channels of accountability and bring confusion in terms of final policy outcomes. Therefore, future policy studies may consider appraising those network configurations that mix different levels and instruments of governance based on criteria of democratic accountability.

In conclusion, much can be learned in the area of network policy making and collaborative governance in Turkish politics and elsewhere in the developing world with benefits for policy practitioners and researchers alike. In the case of Turkey, network analysis may be applied in other areas besides health policy including education policy and migration policy. Education policy is a largely understudied policy area from the governance perspective and would serve as a fertile ground of research due to high levels of policy innovation and institutional transformation witnessed recently. Another area of research conducive to network analysis is migration policy which requires careful scholarly attention due to multiplicity of governmental and non-governmental actors that exceed the national borders within a complex system of multi-level governance. Research in the area of migration, as an example of humanitarian crisis management, is likely to stimulate discussion on the possibility of network collaboration in a policy area characterized by higher levels of conflict compared to domestic social and welfare issues, including health policy. Finally, systematic research across policy settings and country cases will not only help researchers interpret findings in varying contexts but will also contribute to theory building efforts on the topic of network collaboration.

Appendix

A. Sample of Organizations Selected for Semi-Structured Interviews

1. *T.C. Sağlık Bakanlığı, Sağlığın Geliştirilmesi Genel Müdürlüğü, Sağlık Turizmi Daire Başkanlığı (Ministry of Health, General Directorate of Health Promotion, Department Health Tourism)*
2. T.C. Sağlık Bakanlığı, *Sağlık Yatırımları Genel Müdürlüğü (Ministry of Health, General Directorate of Health Investments)*
3. T.C. Sağlık Bakanlığı, *Sağlık Yatırımları Genel Müdürlüğü, Kamu Özel İşbirliği Daire Başkanlığı (Ministry of Health, General Directorate of Health Investments, Department of Public-Private Partnerships)*
4. T.C. Sağlık Bakanlığı, *Sağlık Yatırımları Genel Müdürlüğü, Yatırım Modelleri Daire Başkanlığı (Ministry of Health, General Directorate of Health Investments, Department of Investment Models)*
5. T.C. Sağlık Bakanlığı, Türkiye Halk Sağlığı Kurumu, Çevre Sağlığı Daire Başkanlığı (Ministry of Health, Public Health Institute, Department of Environmental Health)
6. T.C. Sağlık Bakanlığı, İlaç ve Tıbbi Cihaz Kurumu (The Ministry of Health, Pharmaceuticals and Medical Devices Agency)
7. T.C. Sağlık Bakanlığı, Türkiye Halk Sağlığı Kurumu, Ankara Halk Sağlığı Müdürlüğü (Ministry of Health, Public Health Institute, Ankara Provincial Directorate of Public Health)
8. T.C. Sağlık Bakanlığı, Ankara İl Sağlığı Müdürlüğü, Halk Sağlığı şube Müdürlüğü (Ministry of Health, Ankara Provincial Health Directorate, Department of Public Health)
9. *T.C. Aile ve Sosyal Politikalar Bakanlığı, Engelli ve Yaşlı Hizmetleri Genel Müdürlüğü/Eğitim, Rehabilitasyon ve Sosyal Hayata Katılım Daire Başkanlığı (Ministry of Family and Social Policies, General Directorate of Services for Disabled and Elderly People/Department of Education, Rehabilitation, and Social Inclusion)*
10. T.C. Kalkınma Bakanlığı, Sağlık ve Sosyal Güvenlik Daire Başkanlığı (Ministry of Development, Department of Health and Social Security)
11. *Batı Akdeniz Kalkınma Ajansı (West Mediterranean Development Agency)*
12. *Çukurova Kalkınma Ajansı (Çukurova Development Agency)*
13. *Dış Ekonomik İlişkiler Kurulu,* Sağlık İş Konseyi *(Foreign Economic Relations Board Health Business Council)*
14. Tum Tıbbi Cihaz Üretici ve Tedarikçi Federasyonu *(Federation of Medical Device Manufacturers and Suppliers)*
15. *Türkiye Aile Sağlığı ve Planlanması Vakfi (Family Health and Planning Foundations of Turkey)*

16. *Türkiye Sağlık Endüstrisi İşverenler (Healthcare Industry Employers Association)*
17. *Türkiye Sağlık Turizmini Geliştirme Konseyi Derneği (Turkish Healthcare Tourism Development Council)*
18. *Dışkapı Eğitim ve Araştırma Hastanesi, Aile Hekimliği Kliniği (Dışkapı Education and Research Hospital, Family Health Clinic)*
19. Karadeniz Teknik Üniversitesi, Halk Sağlığı Anabilim Dalı (Karadeniz Technical University, Public Health Department)
20. *Evde Bakım Derneği (Home Care Association of Turkey)*
21. *Evde Sağlık ve Sosyal Hizmetler Derneği, EVSAD (Home Healthcare and Social Services Association)*
22. Kanıta Dayalı Tıp Derneği (Evidence-Based Health Association)
23. *Kent Sağlık Grubu (Kent Health Group)*
24. *Ostim Medikal Sanayi Kümelenmesi* (Ostim Medical Industry Cluster*)*
25. *Sağlığın Geliştirilmesi Derneği (Health Development Association)*
26. *Sağlık Turizmi Geliştirme Derneği (Health Tourism Development Association)*

B. Interview Questions and Coding
First Set of Questions

a) Has your organization ever participated in cross-sectoral collaborative projects with any other public, private, or voluntary organizations with the purpose of health policy making? If yes, can you briefly describe the project?
b) In which sub-area(s) of health policy did you collaborate? (a) Public Health, (b) Medical Industry, (c) Health Tourism, (d) Community Health Services, (e) Other

Category 1: Structural Capacity

a) How many other organizations are involved in the collaborative project? Which other organizations have you collaborated with? (a) Public organizations (central/local government), (b) Semi-public organizations/agencies, (c) Private sector organizations (companies/industry associations), (d) Voluntary organizations (professional associations, community-based organizations), (e) Universities (inclusiveness).
b) How frequently do you communicate with representatives of other organizations? Does your interaction take the form of face-to-face communication? (connectedness)
c) At which stage(s) of policy making did you collaborate? (a) Agenda building or identifying policy problems, (b) Policy formulation or designing policy proposals, (c) Policy implementation, (d) Policy evaluation such as assessing the effectiveness of policy including cost-benefit analysis. Did you engage in critical decision-making (common decision-making)?
d) What form does collaboration take? Answers include items such as (a) sub-contracting, (b) multi-stake holder consultation meeting, (c) expert workshop with some level of common decision-making in the form of evidence-based

policy making, (d) cross-sectoral project based on co-investment, and (e) cross-sectoral project based on co-investment with co-funding. The level of resource pooling is put in an increasing order. (Interdependence/resource pooling)

e) Do all participants agree on the terms and conditions of the collaborative project from the start? Have any measures been taken in cases when the terms of the contract, if any, have been broken? (Interdependence/organizational rules)

f) Do you think all project participants have a chance to voice and promote their own preferences/positions equally during the collaborative process (horizontal coordination)? Answers to this question are put in a descending order from "all the time" to "never."

Category 2: Relational Capacity

a) Are actors willing to work together knowing that they have different goals, strategies, and even incentives to behave opportunistically (goal convergence)?
b) Do actors agree on a shared goal and move towards it in a mutually supportive manner (solidarity)?
c) Do network participants engage in effective/productive team work where tasks and responsibilities are split up and redistributed among actors (team work)?
d) If yes, would you define the team work among network participants as a highly synergetic relationship that involves mutual learning, knowledge exchange and innovation (synergy)?

Category 3: Institutional Capacity

a) Is the cross-sectoral project you mention associated with any prevailing discourses and ideas such as media discourses, EU/WHO discourses, political discourses, or pre-election discourses (prevailing discourses)?
b) Is the cross-sectoral project being supported by key actors such as prominent political leaders (ministers or political party spokespersons) or high level state officials (director general, head of directorate) with decision-making power in the executive (prominent actors)?
c) Is the cross-sectoral project aligned with a political coalition, business-based alliance or any other already existing and long-standing web of relations (presence of political coalitions or business-based alliances)?
d) Are there formal institutions or relevant legislation concerning the policy area under investigation (legislation and government departments)?

References

Abimbola, S., Negin, J., Martiniuk, A. L., & Jan, S. (2017). Institutional analysis of health system governance. *Health Policy and Planning*, *32*(9), 1337–1344.

Ağar, A., & Sørensen, E. (2018). Managing collaborative innovation in public bureaucracies. *Planning Theory*, *17*(1), 53–73.

Ağartan, T. (2005). Health sector reform in Turkey: Old policies new politics. In *ESPANET Young researchers workshop*. Retrieved from https://www.academia.edu/7264044/Health_Sector_Reform_in_Turkey_Old_Policies_New_Politics

Ağartan, T. I. (2012). Marketization and universalism: Crafting the right balance in the Turkish healthcare system. *Current Sociology*, *60*(4), 456–471.

Ağartan, T. I. (2015). Health workforce policy and Turkey's health care reform. *Health Policy*, *119*(12), 1621–1626.

Ağartan, T. I. (2016). Learn, frame and deploy? Cross-national policy ideas and comparisons in Turkey's health reform. *Journal of Comparative Policy Analysis: Research and Practice*, *18*(1), 54–69.

Agranoff, R. (2006). Inside collaborative networks: Ten lessons for public managers. *Public Administration Review*, *66*(1), 56–65.

Agranoff, R., & McGuire, M. (1999). Managing in network settings. *Review of Policy Research*, *16*(1), 18–41.

Agranoff, R., & McGuire, M. (2001). Big questions in public network management research. *Journal of Public Administration Research and Theory*, *11*(3), 295–326.

Agranoff, R., & Yıldız, M. (2007). Decision-making in public management networks. In G. Morcol (Ed.), *Handbook of decision-making* (pp. 319–343). New York, NY: Taylor & Francis.

Akbulut, Y., Sarp, N., & Uğurluoğlu, E. (2007). Reform of the health care system in Turkey: A review of universal health insurance. *World Hospitals and Health Services*, *43*(1), 13.

Akça, İ., Bekmen, A., & Özden, B. A. (Eds.). (2014). *Turkey reframed: Constituting neoliberal hegemony*. London: Pluto Press.

Akdağ, R. (2015). Lessons from health transformation in Turkey: Leadership and challenges. *Health Systems & Reform*, *1*(1), 3–8.

Akıncı, F., Mollahaliloğlu, S., Gürsöz, H., & Öğücü, F. (2012). Assessment of the Turkish health care system reforms: A stakeholder analysis. *Health Policy*, *107*(1), 21–30.

Aktulay, G. (1996). *Health Care systems in Transition: Turkey*. Copenhagen: WHO Regional Office for Europe.

Alexander, J., Nank, R., & Stivers, C. (1999). Implications of welfare reform: Do nonprofit survival strategies threaten civil society? *Nonprofit and Voluntary Sector Quarterly*, *28*(4), 452–475.

Alper, Y. (2011). Sosyal güvenlik reformu ve finansmanla ilgili beklentiler. *SGD-Sosyal Güvenlik Dergisi*, *1*(1), 7–47.

Ansell, C., & Gash, A. (2008). Collaborative governance in theory and practice. *Journal of Public Administration Research and Theory*, *18*(4), 543–571.

Aran, M., & Rokx, C. (2014). *Turkey on the way of universal health coverage through the Health Transformation Program (2003–2013)* (No. 91326). Washington, DC: The World Bank.

Assens, C., & Lemeur, A. C. (2016). *Networks governance, partnership management and coalitions federation*. New York, NY: Springer.

Ataay, F. (2008). Sağlık reformu ve yurttaşlık hakları. Amme İdaresi Dergisi, *41*(3), 169–184.

Ataay, F. (2018). Kamu-özel işbirliği modeli üzerine eleştirel bir değerlendirme: Sağlık sektörü örneği. *Ouo Vadis: Kamu Yönetimi*, 403–416.

Atiyas, İ., & Bakış, O. (2015). Structural change and industrial policy in Turkey. *Emerging Markets Finance and Trade*, *51*(6), 1209–1229.

Atkinson, M. M., & Coleman, W. D. (1989). Strong states and weak states: Sectoral policy networks in advanced capitalist economies. *British Journal of Political Science*, *19*(1), 47–67.

Atun, R., Aydın, S., Chakraborty, S., Sümer, S., Aran, M., Gürol, I., & Akdağ, R. (2013). Universal health coverage in Turkey: Enhancement of equity. *The Lancet*, *382*(9886), 65–99.

Axelsson, R., & Axelsson, S. B. (2006). Integration and collaboration in public health: A conceptual framework. *The International Journal of Health Planning and Management*, *21*(1), 75–88.

Aytaç, S. E. (2014). Distributive politics in a multiparty system: The conditional cash transfer program in Turkey. *Comparative Political Studies*, *47*(9), 1211–1237.

Bardach, E. (1998). *Getting agencies to work together: The practice and theory of managerial craftsmanship*. Washington, DC: Brookings Institution Press.

Barış, E., Mollahalıloğlu, S., & Aydin, S. (2011). Healthcare in Turkey: From laggard to leader. *BMJ*, *342*, c7456.

Basu, S., Andrews, J., Kishore, S., Panjabi, R., & Stuckler, D. (2012). Comparative performance of private and public healthcare systems in low-and middle-income countries: A systematic review. *PLoS Medicine*, *9*(6), e1001244.

Baumgartner, F., & Jones, B. (2009). *Agendas and instability in American politics* (2nd ed.). Chicago, IL: The University of Chicago Press.

Baumgartner, F. R., Breunig, C., Green-Pedersen, C., Jones, B. D., Mortensen, P. B., Nuytemans, M., & Walgrave, S. (2009). Punctuated equilibrium in comparative perspective. *American Journal of Political Science*, *53*(3), 603–620.

Bennett, S., Glandon, D., & Rasanathan, K. (2018). Governing multisectoral action for health in low-income and middle-income countries: Unpacking the problem and rising to the challenge. *BMJ Global Health*, *3*(4), e000880.

Berardo, R. (2009). Generalized trust in multi-organizational policy arenas: Studying its emergence from a network perspective. *Political Research Quarterly*, *62*(1), 178–189.

Berardo, R., & Scholz, J. T. (2010). Self-organizing policy networks: Risk, partner selection, and cooperation in estuaries. *American Journal of Political Science*, *54*(3), 632–649.

Berry, F. S., Brower, R. S., Choi, S. O., Goa, W. X., Jang, H., Kwon, M., & Word, J. (2004). Three traditions of network research: What the public management research agenda can learn from other research communities. *Public Administration Review*, *64*(5), 539–552.

Bertelli, A. M., & Smith, C. R. (2009). Relational contracting and network management. *Journal of Public Administration Research and Theory*, *20*(1), i21–i40.

Best, A., Berland, A., Greenhalgh, T., Bourgeault, I. L., Saul, J. E., & Barker, B. (2018). Networks as systems: A case study of the World Health Organisation's Global Health Workforce Alliance. *Journal of Health Organization and Management*, *32*(1), 9–24.

Bilir, N., Çakır, B., Dağlı, E., Ergüder, T., & Önder, Z. (2009). Tobacco control in Turkey. *WHO Europe*, Retrieved from http://www.euro.who.int/__data/assets/pdf_file/0004/98446/E93038.pdf

Blanco, I., Lowndes, V., & Pratchett, L. (2011). Policy networks and governance networks: Towards greater conceptual clarity. *Political Studies Review*, *9*(3), 297–308.

Blom-Hansen, J. (1997). A 'new institutional' perspective on policy networks. *Public Administration*, *75*(4), 669–693.

Bogason, P., & Toonen, T. A. (1998). Introduction: Networks in public administration. *Public Administration, 76*(2), 205–227.

Bogner, A., Littig, B., & Menz, W. (2009). Introduction: Expert interviews – An introduction to a new methodological debate. In A. Bogner, B. Littig, & W. Menz (Eds.), *Interviewing experts* (pp. 1–13). London: Palgrave Macmillan.

Bölükbaşı, H. T., & Ertuğal, E. (2018). Turkey's statist policy style. *Policy styles and policy making: Exploring the linkages*. Abingdon-on-Thames: Routledge.

Bölükbaşı, H. T., Ertuğal, E., & Özçürümez, S. (2010). The impact of the EU on Turkey: Toward streamlining Europeanisation as a research programme. *European Political Science, 9*(4), 464–480.

Bölükbaşı, T. H., Ertuğal, E., & Özçürümez, S. (2018). "Europeanisation of policy making in Turkey and its limits." In C. Bakır & G. Ertan (Eds.), *Policy analysis in Turkey* (pp. 143–161). Bristol: Bristol University Press.

Boratav, K., Yeldan, E., & Köse, A. (2000). Globalization, distribution and social policy: Turkey, 1980–1998. *CEPA and the New School for Social Research, Working Paper Series, 20*, 113–114.

Börzel, T. (1997). What's so special about policy networks? An exploration of the concept and its usefulness in studying European governance. Retrieved from https://papers.ssrn.com/sol3/papers.cfm?abstract_id=302706

Börzel, T. A. (1998). Organizing Babylon-On the different conceptions of policy networks. *Public Administration, 76*(2), 253–273.

Börzel, T. A. (2011). Networks: Reified metaphor or governance panacea? *Public Administration, 89*(1), 49–63.

Bossert, T. J. (2012). Health systems. *Health Policy and Planning, 27*(1), 8–10.

Brass, D. J., Galaskiewicz, J., Greve, H. R., & Tsai, W. (2004). Taking stock of networks and organizations: A multilevel perspective. *Academy of Management Journal, 47*(6), 795–817.

Brass, J. N. (2012). Blurring boundaries: The integration of NGOs into governance in Kenya. *Governance, 25*(2), 209–235.

Bressers, H. (2009). From public administration to policy networks: Contextual interaction analysis. *Rediscovering Public Law and Public Administration in Comparative Policy Analysis: Tribute to Peter Knoepfel*, 123–142.

Bressers, H., O'Toole, L. J., Jr, & Richardson, J. (1994). Networks as models of analysis: Water policy in comparative perspective. *Environmental Politics, 3*(4), 1–23.

Bryman, A. (2007). Barriers to integrating quantitative and qualitative research. *Journal of Mixed Methods Research, 1*(1), 8–22.

Bryman, A., & Burgess, R. G. (2002). Developments in qualitative data analysis: An introduction. In A. Bryman & B. Burgess (Eds.) *Analyzing qualitative data* (pp. 1–17). London: Routledge.

Bulu, M., & Yalçıntaş M. (2015). Cluster as a development policy tool: The Turkish experience. In M. Yülek (Ed.), *Economic planning and industrial policy in the globalizing economy*. Public Administration, Governance and Globalization (Vol. 13, pp. 331–344). Heidelberg, Germany: Springer.

Cabrera, A., & Cabrera, E. F. (2002). Knowledge-sharing dilemmas. *Organization Studies, 23*(5), 687–710.

Cairney, P., & Oliver, K. (2017). Evidence-based policymaking is not like evidence-based medicine, so how far should you go to bridge the divide between evidence and policy? *Health Research Policy and Systems, 15*(1), 35.

Campos, K. D. P., Norman, C. D., & Jadad, A. R. (2011). Product development public–private partnerships for public health: A systematic review using qualitative data. *Social Science & Medicine, 73*(7), 986–994.

Çetin, A., Tekmen, E. E., Karaahmetoğlu, O., & Torun, M. T. (2016). Kümelenme faaliyetlerinin samsun medikal kümesindeki firma yöneticilerince değerlendirilmesi: Beklentiler ve sonuçlar. *Ege Stratejik Araştırmalar Dergisi, 7*(Özel), 69–92.

Chakraborty, S. (2009). Health systems strengthening lessons from the Turkish experience.

Chaskin, R. J. (2001). Building community capacity a definitional framework and case studies from a comprehensive community initiative. *Urban Affairs Review*, *36*(3), 291–323.

Chen, L., & Feng, L. (2017). Analysis on the critical success factors in Public-Private Partnership (PPP) health projects in China. *Chinese Journal of Health Policy*, *10*(3), 1–6.

Chi, M. T. (1997). Quantifying qualitative analyses of verbal data: A practical guide. *The Journal of the Learning Sciences*, *6*(3), 271–315.

Chow, W. S., & Chan, L. S. (2008). Social network, social trust and shared goals in organizational knowledge sharing. *Information & Management*, *45*(7), 458–465.

Ciccone, D. K., Vian, T., Maurer, L., & Bradley, E. H. (2014). Linking governance mechanisms to health outcomes: a review of the literature in low-and middle-income countries. *Social Science & Medicine*, *117*, 86–95.

Coleman, J. S. (1988). Social capital in the creation of human capital. *American Journal of Sociology*, *94*, s95-s120.

Coleman, W. D., Skogstad, G. D., & Atkinson, M. M. (1996). Paradigm shifts and policy networks: Cumulative change in agriculture. *Journal of Public Policy*, *16*(3), 273–301.

Collins, K. M., Onwuegbuzie, A. J., & Jiao, Q. G. (2006). Prevalence of mixed-methods sampling designs in social science research. *Evaluation & Research in Education*, *19*(2), 83–101.

Considine, M., & Lewis, J. M. (2003). Bureaucracy, network, or enterprise? Comparing models of governance in Australia, Britain, the Netherlands, and New Zealand. *Public Administration Review*, *63*(2), 131–140.

Considine, M., Lewis, J. M., & Alexander, D. (2009). *Networks, innovation and public policy: Politicians, bureaucrats and the pathways to change inside government*. Basingstoke, Hampshire: Springer.

Creswell, J. (1998). *Qualitative inquiry and research design: Choosing among five traditions*. Thousand Oaks, CA: Sage.

Currall, S. C., & Judge, T. A. (1995). Measuring trust between organizational boundary role persons. *Organizational Behavior and Human Decision Processes*, *64*(2), 151–170.

Dal Molin, M., & Masella, C. (2016). Networks in policy, management and governance: A comparative literature review to stimulate future research avenues. *Journal of Management & Governance*, *20*(4), 823–849.

Damgaard, B. (2006). Do policy networks lead to network governing? *Public Administration*, *84*(3), 673–691.

DeLeon, P., & Varda, D. M. (2009). Toward a theory of collaborative policy networks: Identifying structural tendencies. *Policy Studies Journal*, *37*(1), 59–74.

Demiralp, S. (2018). Making winners: Urban transformation and neoliberal populism in Turkey. *The Middle East Journal*, *72*(1), 89–108.

Devlet Planlama Teşkilatı. (1984). Beşinci beş yıllık kalkınma planı (1985–1989), Yayın No: 1974. Retrieved from http://ekutup.dpt.gov.tr/plan/plan5.pdf

Dickerson, C., Grills, N., Henwood, N., Jeffreys, S., & Lankester, T. (2012). The World Health Organization engaging with civil society networks to promote primary health care: A case study. *Global Health Governance*, *6*(1), 1–13.

Döner, P., Özkara, A., & Kahveci, R. (2013). Syrian refugees in Turkey: numbers and emotions. *The Lancet*, *382*(9894), 764.

Dorussen, H., Lenz, H., & Blavoukos, S. (2005). Assessing the reliability and validity of expert interviews. *European Union Politics*, *6*(3), 315–337.

Dowding, K. (1995). Model or metaphor? A critical review of the policy network approach. *Political Studies*, *43*(1), 136–158.

Dowding, K. (2001). There must be end to confusion: Policy networks, intellectual fatigue, and the need for political science methods courses in British universities. *Political Studies*, *49*(1), 89–105.

Dündar, P. E. (2018). Sağlıkta sektörler arası işbirliği: Kanıta dayalı uygulamalar. *Turkiye Klinikleri Public Health-Special Topic*, *4*(2), 82–85.

Dunleavy, P., Margetts, H., Bastow, S., & Tinkler, J. (2006). New public management is dead: Long live digital-era governance. *Journal of Public Administration Research and Theory*, *16*(3), 467–494.

Duyulmus, C. U. (2011). Social security reform in Turkey: Different usages of Europe in shaping the national welfare reform. In P. R. Graziano, S. Jacquot & B. Palier (Eds.), *The EU and the Domestic Politics of Welfare State Reforms* (pp. 280–315). London: Palgrave Macmillan.

Eikenberry, A. M., & Kluver, J. D. (2004). The marketization of the nonprofit sector: Civil society at risk? *Public Administration Review*, *64*(2), 132–140.

Ekmekci, P. E. (2017). Syrian refugees, health and migration legislation in Turkey. *Journal of Immigrant and Minority Health*, *19*(6), 1434–1441.

Emerson, K. (2018). Collaborative governance of public health in low-and middle-income countries: lessons from research in public administration. *BMJ Global Health*, *3*(4), e000381.

Erus, B., & Aktakke, N. (2012). Impact of healthcare reforms on out-of-pocket health expenditures in Turkey for public insurers. *The European Journal of Health Economics*, *13*(3), 337–346.

Esen, B., & Gümüşçü, S. (2016). Rising competitive authoritarianism in Turkey. *Third World Quarterly*, *37*(9), 1581–1606.

Esen, B., & Gümüşçü, S. (2018a). Building a competitive authoritarian regime: State–business relations in the AKP's Turkey. *Journal of Balkan and Near Eastern Studies*, *20*(4), 349–372.

Esen, B., & Gümüşçü, S. (2018b). The perils of "Turkish Presidentialism". *Review of Middle East Studies*, *52*(1), 43–53.

Esen, B., & Yardımcı-Geyikçi, Ş. (2019). An Alternative account of the populist backlash in the United States: A perspective from Turkey. *Political Science & Politics*, *52*(3), 445–450.

Etzkowitz, H., & Zhou, C. (2017). *The triple helix: University–industry–government innovation and entrepreneurship*. New York, NY: Routledge.

Falleti, T. G., & Lynch, J. F. (2009). Context and causal mechanisms in political analysis. *Comparative Political Studies*, *42*(9), 1143–1166.

Fikret Paşa, S., Kabasakal, H., & Bodur, M. (2001). Society, organizations, and leadership in Turkey. *Applied Psychology*, *50*(4), 559–589.

Freeman, R., Griggs, S., & Boaz, A. (2011). The practice of policy making. *Evidence and Policy: A Journal of Research, Debate and Practice*, *7*(2), 127–136.

Freudenberg, N., Eng, E., Flay, B., Parcel, G., Rogers, T., & Wallerstein, N. (1994). Strengthening individual and community capacity to prevent disease and promote health: In search of relevant theories and principles. *Health Education & Behavior*, *22*(3), 290–306.

Fulda, A., Li, Y., & Song, Q. (2012). New strategies of civil society in China: A case study of the network governance approach. *Journal of Contemporary China*, *21*(76), 675–693.

Ganesan, S., & Hess, R. (1997). Dimensions and levels of trust: Implications for commitment to a relationship. *Marketing Letters*, *8*(4), 439–448.

Gastil, J. (1993). *Democracy in small groups: Participation, decision-making, and communication*. Philadelphia, PA: New Society Publishers.

Gebara, M. F., Fatorelli, L., May, P., & Zhang, S. (2014). REDD+ policy networks in Brazil: Constraints and opportunities for successful policy making. *Ecology and Society*, *19*(3).

Genckaya, Ö., Togan, S., Schulz, L., & Karadag, R., (2018). Sustainable Governance Indicators. Turkey Report. Bertelsmann Stiftung. Retrieved from https://www.sgi-network.org/docs/2018/country/SGI2018_Turkey.pdf

Givel, M. (2010). The evolution of the theoretical foundations of punctuated equilibrium theory in public policy. *Review of Policy Research, 27*(2), 187–198.

Glandon, D., Meghani, A., Jessani, N., Qiu, M., & Bennett, S. (2018). Identifying health policy and systems research priorities on multisectoral collaboration for health in low-income and middle-income countries. *BMJ Global Health, 3*(4), e000970.

Green, E. C. (2001). Can qualitative research produce reliable quantitative findings? *Field Methods, 13*(1), 3–19.

Greenaway, J., Salter, B., & Hart, S. (2007). How policy networks can damage democratic health: A case study in the government of governance. *Public Administration, 85*(3), 717–738.

Gulati, R. (1995). Does familiarity breed trust? The implications of repeated ties for contractual choice in alliances. *Academy of Management Journal, 38*(1), 85–112.

Gürakar, E. Ç., & Bircan, T. (2018). Redistributive politics, clientelism, and political patronage under the AKP. In L. Ruiz de Elvira, C. H. Schwarz, & I. Weipert-Fenner (Eds.), *Clientelism and patronage in the Middle East and North Africa: Networks of dependency* (pp. 71–98). New York, NY: Routledge.

Gürsoy, K. (2015). An overview of Turkish healthcare system after Health Transformation Program: Main successes, performance assessment, further challenges, and policy options. *Sosyal Güvence, 0*(7), 83–112.

Hale, W., & Özbudun, E. (2009). *Islamism, democracy and liberalism in Turkey: The case of the AKP*. New York, NY: Routledge.

Hall, C. M., & Jenkins, J. M. (2003). *Tourism and Public Policy*. London: Thomson Learning.

Hancké, B. (2009). *Intelligent research design: A guide for beginning researchers in the social sciences*. Oxford: Oxford University Press.

Hardiman, N. (2006). Politics and social partnership: Flexible network governance. *Economic and Social Review, 37*(3), 343–374.

Haveri, A., Nyholm, I., Roiseland, A. R., & Vabo, I. (2009). Governing collaboration: Practices of meta-governance in Finnish and Norwegian local governments. *Local Government Studies, 35*(5), 539–556.

Hazama, Y. (2015). Health reform and service satisfaction in the poor: Turkey 2003–11. *Turkish Studies, 16*(1), 36–53.

Head, B. W. (2016). Toward more "evidence-informed" policy making? *Public Administration Review, 76*(3), 472–484.

Heper, M. (1993). Political culture as a dimension of compatibility. In M. Heper, A. Öncü, & H. Kramer (Eds.). *Turkey and the west: Changing political and cultural identities* (pp. 1–18). New York, NY: IB Tauris.

Heper, M., & Yıldırım, S. (2011). Revisiting civil society in Turkey. *Southeast European and Black Sea Studies, 11*(1), 1–18.

Herranz, J., Jr. (2007). The multisectoral trilemma of network management. *Journal of Public Administration Research and Theory, 18*(1), 1–31.

Hirschi, C., & Widmer, T. (2010). Policy change and policy stasis: Comparing Swiss foreign policy toward South Africa (1968–94) and Iraq (1990–91). *Policy Studies Journal, 38*(3), 537–563.

Hodge, G. A., & Greve, C. (2007). Public–private partnerships: An international performance review. *Public Administration Review, 67*(3), 545–558.

Hoe, C., Rodriguez, D. C., Üzümcüoğlu, Y., & Hyder, A. A. (2016). "Quitting like a Turk:" How political priority developed for tobacco control in Turkey. *Social Science & Medicine, 165*, 36–45.

Hoe, C., Rodriguez, D. C., Üzümcüoğlu, Y., & Hyder, A. A. (2019). Understanding political priority development for public health issues in Turkey: Lessons from tobacco control and road safety. *Health Research Policy and Systems, 17*(1), 13.

Hope, M., & Raudla, R. (2012). Discursive institutionalism and policy stasis in simple and compound polities: The cases of Estonian fiscal policy and United States climate change policy. *Policy Studies*, *33*(5), 399–418.

Horton, R., & Lo, S. (2013). Turkey's democratic transition to universal health coverage. *The Lancet*, *382*(9886), 3.

Howlett, M. (1991). Policy instruments, policy styles, and policy implementation: National approaches to theories of instrument choice. *Policy Studies Journal*, *19*(2), 1–21.

Howlett, M. (2002). Do networks matter? Linking policy network structure to policy outcomes: Evidence from four Canadian policy sectors 1990–2000. *Canadian Journal of Political Science/Revue Canadienne de Science Politique*, *35*(2), 235–267.

Howlett, M. (2011). *Designing public policies: Principles and instruments*. New York, NY: Routledge.

Howlett, M., & Tosun, J. (Eds.). (2018). *Policy styles and policy making: Exploring the linkages*. Abingdon-on-Thames: Routledge.

Huang, K., & Provan, K. G. (2006). Resource tangibility and patterns of interaction in a publicly funded health and human services network. *Journal of Public Administration Research and Theory*, *17*(3), 435–454.

Huang, K., & Provan, K. G. (2007). Structural embeddedness and organizational social outcomes in a centrally governed mental health services network. *Public Management Review*, *9*(2), 169–189.

İnsel, A. (2003). The AKP and normalizing democracy in Turkey. *The South Atlantic Quarterly*, *102*(2), 293–308.

Isett, K. R., & Provan, K. G. (2005). The evolution of dyadic interorganizational relationships in a network of publicly funded nonprofit agencies. *Journal of Public Administration Research and Theory*, *15*(1), 149–165.

Janowicz, M., & Noorderhaven, N. (2006). 15 Levels of inter-organizational trust: conceptualization and measurement. *Handbook of Trust Research*, 264–279.

Janssen, M., & Helbig, N. (2018). Innovating and changing the policy-cycle: Policy-makers be prepared! *Government Information Quarterly*, *35*(4), 99–105.

Jenkins, J. M., & Henry, G. T. (2016). Dispersed vs. centralized policy governance: The case of state early care and education policy. *Journal of Public Administration Research and Theory*, *26*(4), 709–725.

Johnston, L. M., & Finegood, D. T. (2015). Cross-sector partnerships and public health: Challenges and opportunities for addressing obesity and noncommunicable diseases through engagement with the private sector. *Annual Review of Public Health*, *36*, 255–271.

Jordan, A., Wurzel, R. K., & Zito, A. (2005). The rise of 'new' policy instruments in comparative perspective: Has governance eclipsed government? *Political Studies*, *53*(3), 477–496.

Jordan, G., & Schubert, K. (1992). A preliminary ordering of policy network labels. *European Journal of Political Research*, *21*(1–2), 7–27.

Kadirbeyoğlu, Z. (2017). The impact of power and civic engagement in the decentralized management of natural resources: The case of Turkey. *Public Administration and Development*, *37*(4), 277–291.

Kahveci, R., Koç, E. M., & Küçük, E. Ö. (2017). Health technology assessment in Turkey. *International Journal of Technology Assessment in Health Care*, *33*(3), 402–408.

Kahveci, R., & Meads, C. (2008). Analysis of strengths, weaknesses, opportunities, and threats in the development of a health technology assessment program in Turkey. *International Journal of Technology Assessment in Health Care*, *24*(2), 235–240.

Kapucu, N. (2006). Interagency communication networks during emergencies: Boundary spanners in multiagency coordination. *The American Review of Public Administration*, *36*(2), 207–225.

Karatepe, İ. D. (2016). The State, Islamists, discourses, and bourgeoisie: The construction industry in Turkey. *Research and Policy on Turkey*, *1*(1), 46–62.

Kartal, F. (2009). Privatized citizenship: Transformation of health care policies in Turkey. *Review of Public Administration*, *42*(2), 23–43.

Keast, R., Mandell, M. P., Brown, K., & Woolcock, G. (2004). Network structures: Working differently and changing expectations. *Public Administration Review*, *64*(3), 363–371.

Kenis, P., & Provan, K. G. (2009). Towards an exogenous theory of public network performance. *Public Administration*, *87*(3), 440–456.

Kenis, P., & Schneider, V. (1989). Policy networks as an analytical tool for policy analysis. Conference paper presented at Max Planck Institute, Cologne, 4–5 December.

Kenis, P. N., Marin, B., & Mayntz, R. (1991). The preconditions for policy networks: Some findings from a three-country study on industrial restructuring. *Policy Networks*, 297–330.

Kickbusch, I. (2009). Policy innovations for health. In I. Kickbusch (Ed.) *Policy Innovation for Health* (pp. 1–21). New York, NY: Springer.

Kickert, W. J. M., & Koppenjan, J. F. M. (1997). Public management and network management: An overview. In W. J. M. Kickert, E. H. Klijn, & J.F.M. Koppenjan (Eds.), *Managing complex networks: Strategies for the public sector* (pp. 35–61). London: Sage.

Kilic, B. (2014). Health-care reform in Turkey: Far from perfect. *The Lancet*, *383*(9911), 28–29.

Kim, S., & Lee, H. (2006). The impact of organizational context and information technology on employee knowledge-sharing capabilities. *Public Administration Review*, *66*(3), 370–385.

Kjaer, A. M. (2011). Rhodes' Contribution to governance theory: Praise, criticism and the future governance debate. *Public Administration*, *89*(1), 101–113.

Klijn, E. H. (1996). Analyzing and managing policy processes in complex networks: A theoretical examination of the concept policy network and its problems. *Administration & Society*, *28*(1), 90–119.

Klijn, E. H. (2001). Rules as institutional context for decision-making in networks: The approach to postwar housing districts in two cities. *Administration & Society*, *33*(2), 133–164.

Klijn, E. H., & Koppenjan, J. F. (2000). Public management and policy networks: Foundations of a network approach to governance. *Public Management an International Journal of Research and Theory*, *2*(2), 135–158.

Klijn, E. H., Sierra, V., Ysa, T., Berman, E., Edelenbos, J., & Chen, D. Y. (2016). The influence of trust on network performance in Taiwan, Spain, and the Netherlands: A cross-country comparison. *International Public Management Journal*, *19*(1), 111–139.

Klijn, E. H., & Skelcher, C. (2007). Democracy and governance networks: Compatible or not? *Public Administration*, *85*(3), 587–608.

Klijn, E. H., Steijn, B., & Edelenbos, J. (2010). The impact of network management on outcomes in governance networks. *Public Administration*, *88*(4), 1063–1082.

Knill, C., & Lehmkuhl, D. (2002). Private actors and the state: Internationalization and changing patterns of governance. *Governance* *15*(1), 41–63.

Knox, H., Savage, M., & Harvey, P. (2006). Social networks and the study of relations: Networks as method, metaphor and form. *Economy and Society*, *35*(1), 113–140.

Köse, I., Akpınar, N., Gürel, M., Arslan, Y., Özer, H., Yurt, N., & Dogac, A. (2008). Turkey's national health information system (NHIS). In *The proceedings of the e-Challenges 2008 conference*, Stockholm (pp. 170–177). Retrieved from https://www.srdc.com.tr/share/publications/2008/9.pdf

Kraak, V. I., & Story, M. (2010). A public health perspective on healthy lifestyles and public–private partnerships for global childhood obesity prevention. *Journal of the Academy of Nutrition and Dietetics*, *110*(2), 192–200.

Laws, D., & Hajer, M. (2006). Policy in practice. In R. E. Goodin, M. Moran, & M. Rein (Eds.), *The Oxford handbook of public policy* (pp. 409–424). Oxford: Oxford University Press.

Lecy, J. D., Mergel, I. A., & Schmitz, H. P. (2014). Networks in public administration: Current scholarship in review. *Public Management Review*, *16*(5), 643–665.

Lehoux, P., Denis, J. L., Tailliez, S., & Hivon, M. (2005). Dissemination of health technology assessments: Identifying the visions guiding an evolving policy innovation in Canada. *Journal of Health Politics, Policy and Law*, *30*(4), 603–642.

Levine, S., & White, P. E. (1961). Exchange as a conceptual framework for the study of interorganizational relationships. *Administrative Science Quarterly*, 583–601.

Lewis, J. M. (2006). Being around and knowing the players: Networks of influence in health policy. *Social Science & Medicine*, *62*(9), 2125–2136.

Lewis, J. M. (2011). The future of network governance research: Strength in diversity and synthesis. *Public Administration*, *89*(4), 1221–1234.

Littig, B. (2009). Interviewing the elite: Interviewing experts: Is there a difference? In A. Bogner, B. Littig, & W. Menz (Eds.), *Interviewing experts* (pp. 98–113). London: Palgrave Macmillan.

Lowi, T. J. (1972). Four systems of policy, politics, and choice. *Public Administration Review*, *32*(4), 298–310.

Lowndes, V. (2001). Rescuing Aunt Sally: Taking institutional theory seriously in urban politics. *Urban Studies*, *38*(11), 1953–1971.

Lowndes, V., & Roberts, M. (2013). *Why institutions matter: The new institutionalism in political science*. London: Macmillan International Higher Education.

Lundin, M. (2007). Explaining cooperation: How resource interdependence, goal congruence, and trust affect joint actions in policy implementation. *Journal of Public Administration Research and Theory*, *17*(4), 651–672.

Mahoney, J., & Goertz, G. (2004). The possibility principle: Choosing negative cases in comparative research. *American Political Science Review*, *98*(4), 653–669.

Mandell, M. P. (1999). Community collaborations. *Review of Policy Research*, *16*(1), 42–64.

Marin, B., & Mayntz, R. (1991). *Policy networks: Empirical evidence and theoretical considerations*. Frankfurt, Germany: Campus Verlag.

Marsh, D., & Smith, M. (2000). Understanding policy networks: Towards a dialectical approach. *Political Studies*, *48*(1), 4–21.

Martsolf, G. R., Sloan, J., Villarruel, A., Mason, D., & Sullivan, C. (2018). Promoting a culture of health through cross-sector collaborations. *Health Promotion Practice*, *19*(5), 784–791.

Mason, J. (2002). *Qualitative researching*. Thousand Oaks, CA: Sage.

Mattessich, P. W., & Rausch, E. J. (2014). Cross-sector collaboration to improve community health: A view of the current landscape. *Health Affairs*, *33*(11), 1968–1974.

Mayntz, R. (1993). Modernization and the logic of interorganizational networks. *Knowledge and Policy*, *6*(1), 3–16.

McGuire, M. (2006). Collaborative public management: Assessing what we know and how we know it. *Public Administration Review*, *66*(1), 33–43.

McGuire, M., & Agranoff, R. (2011). The limitations of public management networks. *Public Administration*, *89*(2), 265–284.

McKenzie, B. (2015). PPP in Turkey: Turkey reforms healthcare PPPs to encourage investment. Retrieved from https://ceelegalmatters.com/index.php/over-the-wire/legal-ticker-deals-and-cases-in-cee/item/2121-magnusson-advises-octava-on-real-estate-acquisitions-in-poland

Milward, H. B., Provan, K. G., Fish, A., Isett, K. R., & Huang, K. (2009). Governance and collaboration: An evolutionary study of two mental health networks. *Journal of Public Administration Research and Theory*, *20*(suppl_1), i125–i141.

Meyer, E., & Scheepers, C. (2017). Contextual leadership of a multi-partner approach to health care innovation. *Emerald Emerging Markets Case Studies*, *7*(1), 1–29.

Mindlin, Y. B., Zhukov, B. M., Prokhorova, V. V., Shutilov, F. V., & Belova, E. O. (2016). Main stages of the formation of an economic cluster. *International Journal of Economics and Financial Issues*, *6*(1S), 261–265.

Ministry of Development. (2017). *Kamu-özel işbirliği uygulamalarında etkin yönetim.* 11. Kalkınma Planı (2019–2023) Kamu Özel İşbirliği Özel Ihtisas Komisyonu Ön Raporu. Retrieved from http://onbirinciplan.gov.tr/wp-content/uploads/2018/01/Kamu-%C3%96zel-%C4%B0%C5%9Fbirli%C4%9Fi-Uygulamalar%C4%B1nda-Etkin-Y%C3%B6netim-%C3%96n-Rapor.pdf

Ministry of Health. (2009). *Ministry of Health of Turkey Strategic Plan 2010–2014.* Ankara. Retrieved from https://dosyasb.saglik.gov.tr/Eklenti/538,saglik-bakanligi-2010-2014-stratejik-eylem-planipdf.pdf?0

Ministry of Health (2010). *Health Statistics Yearbook.* Retrieved from https://dosyasb.saglik.gov.tr/Eklenti/5102,saglikistatistikleriyilligi2010pdf.pdf?0. Accessed on Accessed on March 25, 2019.

Ministry of Health. (2012). *Ministry of Health of Turkey Strategic Plan 2013–2017.* Ankara. Retrieved from https://sgb.saglik.gov.tr/Dkmanlar/Strategic%20Plan%202013-2017.pdf. Accessed on June 25, 2019.

Ministry of Health. (2013). *Evaluation report on medical tourism in Turkey.* Republic of Turkey Ministry of Health, Directorate General of Health Services, Department of Health Tourism. Retrieved from https://saglik.gov.tr/Eklenti/468,evaluaton-report-on-medical-tourism-in-turkey-2013pdf.pdf?0

Ministry of Health. (2013). *Policy declaration.* Health Technology Assessment Department: General Directorate of Health Research. Retrieved from http://www.hta.gov.tr/EN/pdf/politika.pdf

Ministry of Health. (2014). *Çok sektörlü sağlık sorumluluğunu geliştirme programı* (2013 – 2023). Türkiye Halk Sağlığı Kurumu/Turkish Institute of Public Health. Ankara. Retrievedfrom:https://hsgm.saglik.gov.tr/depo/birimler/cevre-sagligi/1-su-guvenligi/Kitaplar/CokPaydaslisaglsorgelisProOzet_Kitap.pdf

Ministry of Health. (2017). *Multisectoral action plan on noncommunicable diseases (2017–2025).* Ministry of Health Publication Number 1057. Ankara. Retrieved from http://www.euro.who.int/__data/assets/pdf_file/0005/346694/BOH_ENG.pdf?ua=1

Mitton, C., Adair, C. E., McKenzie, E., Patten, S. B., & Perry, B. W. (2007). Knowledge transfer and exchange: review and synthesis of the literature. *The Milbank Quarterly*, *85*(4), 729–768.

Morse, J. M. (1994). Designing qualitative research. In N. K. Denzin & Y. S. Lincoln (Eds.), *Handbook of qualitative inquiry* (pp. 220–235). Thousand Oaks, CA: Sage.

Morse, J. M. (2000). Determining sample size. *Qualitative Health Research*, *10*(1), 3–5.

Moser, S. C., & Dilling, L. (2007). Toward the social tipping point: Creating a climate for change. *Creating a climate for change: Communicating climate change and facilitating social change* (pp. 491–516). Cambridge: Cambridge University Press.

Murthy, K. J. R., Frieden, T. R., Yazdani, A., & Hreshikesh, P. (2001). Public–private partnership in tuberculosis control: Experience in Hyderabad, India. *The International Journal of Tuberculosis and Lung Disease*, *5*(4), 354–359.

Nederhand, J., & Klijn, E. H. (2019). Stakeholder involvement in public–private partnerships: Its influence on the innovative character of projects and on project performance. *Administration & Society*, *51*(8), 1200–1226.

O'Toole, L. J., Jr. (1997). Treating networks seriously: Practical and research-based agendas in public administration. *Public Administration Review*, 45–52.

O'Toole, L. J., Jr. (2003). Interorganizational relations in implementation. In B. G. Peters & J. Pierre (Eds.), *Handbook of public administration* (pp. 234–244). London: Sage Publications.

Ocaklı, F. (2018). Reconfiguring state–business relations in Turkey: Housing and hydroelectric energy sectors in comparative perspective. *Journal of Balkan and Near Eastern Studies*, *20*(4), 373–387.

OECD/The World Bank. (2008). *OECD Reviews of Health Systems-Turkey*. Paris: OECD Publishing. Retrieved from https://www.oecd-ilibrary.org/social-issues-migration-health/oecd-reviews-of-health-systems-turkey-2008_9789264051096-en

OECD (2017). Better Life Index Database, Retrieved from www.oecdbetterlifeindex.org.

Ökem, Z. G., & Çakar, M. (2015). What have health care reforms achieved in Turkey? An appraisal of the "Health Transformation Programme." *Health Policy*, *119*(9), 1153–1163.

Öktem, K., & Akkoyunlu, K. (2016). Exit from democracy: Illiberal governance in Turkey and beyond. *Southeast European and Black Sea Studies*, *16*(4), 469–480.

Olsen, J. P. (2005). Maybe it is time to rediscover bureaucracy. *Journal of Public Administration Research and Theory*, *16*(1), 1–24.

Öncü, T. S. (2017). Verimsiz ve pahalı bir finansman modeli: Kamu-özel ortaklığı. *Şehir Hastaneleri Sempozyumu (bildiri kitabı)*, 52–66.

Öniş, Z. (2019). Turkey under the challenge of state capitalism: The political economy of the late AKP era. *Southeast European and Black Sea Studies*, 1–25.

Onwuegbuzie, A. J., & Leech, N. L. (2007). A call for qualitative power analyses. *Quality & Quantity*, *41*(1), 105–121.

Özbudun, E. (2014). AKP at the crossroads: Erdoğan's majoritarian drift. *South European Society and Politics*, *19*(2), 155–167.

Özbudun, E. (2015). Turkey's judiciary and the drift toward competitive authoritarianism. *The International Spectator*, *50*(2), 42–55.

Özçetin, B., & Özer, M. (2015). The current policy environment for civil society in Turkey (No. 53). Working Papers of the Johns Hopkins Comparative Non Profit Sector Project. Retrieved from http://ccss.jhu.edu/wpcontent/uploads/downloads/2015/02/Turkey_CNP_WP53_2015_FINAL.pdf

Özçevik, O., Beygo, C., & Akçakaya, I. (2010). Building capacity through collaborative local action: Case of Matra REGIMA within Zeytinburnu regeneration scheme. *Journal of Urban Planning and Development*, *136*(2), 169–175.

Özkan, S. (2018). Türkiye'de sağlıkta sektörler arası işbirliği. *Turkiye Klinikleri Public Health-Special Topic*, *4*(2), 86–91.

Paker, H., Adaman, F., Kadirbeyoğlu, Z., & Özkaynak, B. (2013). Environmental organisations in Turkey: Engaging the state and capital. *Environmental Politics*, *22*(5), 760–778.

Pala, K. (2018). Yerel yönetimlerde sağlıkta sektörler arası işbirliği. *Turkiye Klinikleri Public Health-Special Topic*, *4*(2), 92–98.

Park, H. H., & Rethemeyer, R. K. (2012). The politics of connections: Assessing the determinants of social structure in policy networks. *Journal of Public Administration Research and Theory*, *24*(2), 349–379.

Parker, R. (2007). Networked governance or just networks? Local governance of the knowledge economy in Limerick (Ireland) and Karlskrona (Sweden). *Political Studies*, *55*(1), 113–132.

Peters, D. T., Klijn, E. H., Stronks, K., & Harting, J. (2017). Policy coordination and integration, trust, management and performance in public health-related policy networks: a survey. *International Review of Administrative Sciences*, *83*(1), 200–222.

Pierson, P. (2000). Increasing returns, path dependence, and the study of politics. *American Political Science Review*, *94*(2), 251–267.

Porter, M. E. (1998). Clusters and the new economics of competition. *Harvard Business Review*, *76*(6), 77–90.

Provan, K. G., Huang, K., & Milward, H. B. (2009). The evolution of structural embeddedness and organizational social outcomes in a centrally governed health and human services network. *Journal of Public Administration Research and Theory, 19*(4), 873–893.

Provan, K. G., Isett, K. R., & Milward, H. B. (2004). Cooperation and compromise: A network response to conflicting institutional pressures in community mental health. *Nonprofit and Voluntary Sector Quarterly, 33*(3), 489–514.

Provan, K. G., & Kenis, P. (2008). Modes of network governance: Structure, management, and effectiveness. *Journal of Public Administration Research and Theory, 18*(2), 229–252.

Provan, K. G., & Milward, H. B. (1995). A preliminary theory of interorganizational network effectiveness: A comparative study of four community mental health systems. *Administrative Science Quarterly*, 1–33.

Provan, K. G., & Milward, H. B. (1999). Do networks really work? A framework for evaluating public-sector organizational networks. *Academy of Management Proceedings, 1999*(1), A1–A6.

Provan, K. G., & Milward, H. B. (2001). Do networks really work? A framework for evaluating public-sector organizational networks. *Public Administration Review, 61*(4), 414–423.

Provan, K. G., Milward, H. B., & Isett, K. R. (2002). Collaboration and integration of community-based health and human services in a nonprofit managed care system. *Health Care Management Review, 27*(1), 21–32.

Pyone, T., Smith, H., & van den Broek, N. (2017). Frameworks to assess health systems governance: a systematic review. *Health Policy and Planning, 32*(5), 710–722.

Raab, J. (2002). Where do policy networks come from? *Journal of Public Administration Research and Theory, 12*(4), 581–622.

Raab, J., & Milward, H. B. (2003). Dark networks as problems. *Journal of Public Administration Research and Theory, 13*(4), 413–439.

Rasanathan, K., Atkins, V., Mwansambo, C., Soucat, A., & Bennett, S. (2018). Governing multisectoral action for health in low-income and middle-income countries: an agenda for the way forward. *BMJ Global Health, 3*(4), e000890.

Rayner, J., Howlett, M., Wilson, J., Cashore, B., & Hoberg, G. (2001). Privileging the sub-sector: Critical sub-sectors and sectoral relationships in forest policy making. *Forest Policy and Economics, 2*(3–4), 319–332.

Reich, M. R. (2002). *Public–private partnerships for public health*. Harvard Series on Population and International Health. Cambridge, MA: Harvard University Press.

Rethemeyer, R. K., & Hatmaker, D. M. (2007). Network management reconsidered: An inquiry into management of network structures in public sector service provision. *Journal of Public Administration Research and Theory, 18*(4), 617–646.

Rhodes, R. A., & Marsh, D. (1992). New directions in the study of policy networks. *European Journal of Political Research, 21*(1–2), 181–205.

Rhodes, R. A. W. (1990). Policy networks: A British perspective. *Journal of Theoretical Politics, 2*(3), 293–317.

Rhodes, R. A. W. (1996). The new governance: Governing without government. *Political Studies, 44*(4), 652–667.

Rhodes, R. A. W. (1997). *Understanding governance: Policy networks, governance, reflexivity and accountability*. Philadelphia, PA: Open University Press.

Rhodes, R. A. W. (2007). Understanding governance: Ten years on. *Organization Studies, 28*(8), 1243–1264.

Richardson, J. (2000). Government, interest groups and policy change. *Political Studies, 48*(5), 1006–1025.

Richardson, J. (2012). New governance or old governance? A policy style perspective. In D. Levi-Faur (Ed.), *The Oxford handbook of governance* (pp. 311–324). Oxford: Oxford University Press.

Ritchie, J., & Spencer, L. (2002). Qualitative data analysis for applied policy research. In A. Bryman & B. Burgess (Eds.), *Analyzing qualitative data* (pp. 173–194). London: Routledge.

Roberts, N. C., & King, P. J. (1991). Policy entrepreneurs: Their activity structure and function in the policy process. *Journal of Public Administration Research and Theory*, *1*(2), 147–175.

Robichau, R. W. (2011). The mosaic of governance: Creating a picture with definitions, theories, and debates. *Policy Studies Journal*, *39*(1), 113–131.

Rose, R., & Mackenzie, W. J. M. (1991). Comparing forms of comparative analysis. *Political Studies*, *39*(3), 446–462.

Rosenfeld, S. A. (1997). Bringing business clusters into the mainstream of economic development. *European Planning Studies*, *5*(1), 3–23.

Roussos, S. T., & Fawcett, S. B. (2000). A review of collaborative partnerships as a strategy for improving community health. *Annual Review of Public Health*, *21*(1), 369–402.

Rycroft-Malone, J., Burton, C. R., Bucknall, T., Graham, I. D., Hutchinson, A. M., & Stacey, D. (2016). Collaboration and co-production of knowledge in healthcare: Opportunities and challenges. *International Journal of Health Policy and Management*, *5*(4), 221.

Sabel, C. F., & Simon, W. H. (2012). Contextualizing regimes: Institutionalization as a response to the limits of interpretation and policy engineering, *Michigan Law Review*. Columbia Law School, *110*(7), 1265–1309.

Sahin, I., Özcan, Y. A., & Özgen, H. (2011). Assessment of hospital efficiency under Health Transformation Program in Turkey. *Central European Journal of Operations Research*, *19*(1), 19–37.

Sanderson, I. (2002). Evaluation, policy learning and evidence-based policy making. *Public Administration*, *80*(1), 1–22.

Savaş, B. S., Karahan, O. & Saka, R. O (2002). Health care systems in transition: Turkey. Retrieved from http://www.euro.who.int/__data/assets/pdf_file/0007/96415/e79838.pdf

Sayarı, S. (2014). Interdisciplinary approaches to political clientelism and patronage in Turkey. *Turkish Studies*, *15*(4), 655–670.

Sayari, S., & Esmer, Y. R. (Eds.). (2002). *Politics, parties, and elections in Turkey*. Boulder, CO: Lynne Rienner Publishers.

Scharpf, F. W., & Mohr, M. (1994). *Efficient self-coordination in policy networks: A simulation study*. MPIfG Discussion Paper 94/1, Max Planck Institute for the Study of Societies. Retrieved from https://www.econstor.eu/bitstream/10419/43733/1/043523781.pdf

Schwartz, J. B., & Bhushan, I. (2004). Improving immunization equity through a public–private partnership in Cambodia. *Bulletin of the World Health Organization*, *82*, 661–667.

Seawright, J., & Gerring, J. (2008). Case selection techniques in case study research: A menu of qualitative and quantitative options. *Political Research Quarterly*, *61*(2), 294–308.

Shiroma, E. O. (2014). Networks in action: New actors and practices in education policy in Brazil. *Journal of Education Policy*, *29*(3), 323–348.

Shrestha, M. K. (2012). Self-organizing network capital and the success of collaborative public programs. *Journal of Public Administration Research and Theory*, *23*(2), 307–329.

Siddiqi, S., Masud, T. I., Nishtar, S., Peters, D. H., Sabri, B., Bile, K. M., & Jama, M. A. (2009). Framework for assessing governance of the health system in developing countries: Gateway to good governance. *Health Policy*, *90*(1), 13–25.

Skilling, M. D. (2015). Dispute resolution in the health sector PPPs: The Turkish Experience BASEAK White Papers: December 2015, No: 4. Retrieved from https://

www.baseak.com/en/insights/reports-and-whitepapers/2016/may/26/dispute-resolution-in-the-health-sector-ppps?ParentItemID=440ymEOm1qNzuDAToZ1rUlHcgNNN0csAQG2FaHooIOVWFCm9GbPdkA==&Archive=False

Somer, M. (2016). Understanding Turkey's democratic breakdown: old vs. new and indigenous vs. global authoritarianism. *Southeast European and Black Sea Studies*, *16*(4), 481–503.

Sørensen, E. (2002). Democratic theory and network governance. *Administrative Theory & Praxis*, *24*(4), 693–720.

Sørensen, E. (2005). The democratic problems and potentials of network governance. *European Political Science*, *4*(3), 348–357.

Sørensen, E. (2006). Metagovernance: The changing role of politicians in processes of democratic governance. *The American Review of Public Administration*, *36*(1), 98–114.

Sørensen, E., & Torfing, J. (2005). The democratic anchorage of governance networks. *Scandinavian Political Studies*, *28*(3), 195–218.

Sørensen, E., & Torfing, J. (2007). *Theories of democratic network governance*. Basingstoke: Palgrave Macmillan.

Sørensen, E., & Torfing, J. (2009). Making governance networks effective and democratic through metagovernance. *Public Administration*, *87*(2), 234–258.

Sørensen, E., & Torfing, J. (2016). Metagoverning collaborative innovation in governance networks. *The American Review of Public Administration*, *47*(7), 826–839.

Sparkes, S. P., Bump, J. B., & Reich, M. R. (2015). Political strategies for health reform in Turkey: Extending veto point theory. *Health Systems & Reform*, *1*(4), 263–275.

Stoker, G. (1998). Governance as theory: Five propositions. *International Social Science Journal*, *50*(155), 17–28.

Stoker, G. (2006). Public value management: A new narrative for networked governance? *The American Review of Public Administration*, *36*(1), 41–57.

Sülkü, S. N. (2011). The health sector reforms and the efficiency of public hospitals in Turkey: Provincial markets. *The European Journal of Public Health*, *22*(5), 634–638.

Sullivan, H., & Skelcher, C. (2017). *Working across boundaries: Collaboration in public services*. London: Macmillan International Higher Education.

Swanson, R. C., Atun, R., Best, A., Betigeri, A., de Campos, F., Chunharas, S., & Omaswa, F. (2015). Strengthening health systems in low-income countries by enhancing organizational capacities and improving institutions. *Globalization and Health*, *11*(1), 5.

Tangcharoensathien, V., Srisookwatana, O., Pinprateep, P., Posayanonda, T., & Patcharanarumol, W. (2017). Multisectoral actions for health: Challenges and opportunities in complex policy environments. *International Journal of Health Policy and Management*, *6*(7), 359–363.

Tansel, C. B. (2018). Authoritarian neoliberalism and democratic backsliding in Turkey: Beyond the narratives of progress. *South European Society and Politics*, *23*(2), 197–217.

Tatar, M., & Kanavos, P. (2006). Health care reform in Turkey. *EUROHEALTH-LONDON-*, *12*(1), 20.

Tatar, M., Mollahaliloğlu, S., Şahin, B., Aydın, S., Maresso, A., & Hernández-Quevedo, C. (2011). Turkey. Health system review. *Health Systems in Transition*, *13*(6), 1–186. Retrieved from http://www.euro.who.int/__data/assets/pdf_file/0006/158883/e96441.pdf

Tekin, P. Ş., & Çelik, Y. (2010). Türkiye'de sağlık sektöründe bir finansman yöntemi olarak kamu-özel ortaklığı politikasının politika haritalama yöntemi ile analiz edilmesi. *Ankara Sağlık Bilimleri Dergisi*, *1*(3), 81–98.

Tenbensel, T., Cumming, J., Ashton, T., & Barnett, P. (2008). Where there's a will, is there a way? Is New Zealand's publicly funded health sector able to steer towards population health? *Social Science & Medicine*, *67*(7), 1143–1152.

Tenbensel, T., Mays, N., & Cumming, J. (2011). A successful mix of hierarchy and collaboration? Interpreting the 2001 reform of the governance of the New Zealand public health system. *Policy & Politics*, *39*(2), 239–255.

Timur, S., & Getz, D. (2008). A network perspective on managing stakeholders for sustainable urban tourism. *International Journal of Contemporary Hospitality Management*, *20*(4), 445–461.

TMA. (2011). *Sağlıkta hayaller, yalanlar ve gerçekler*. (*Illusions, lies and truth in healthcare*.) Ankara, Turkey: TMA Publications.

TMMOB/ATO. (2017). *Şehir Hastaneleri sempozyumu*. (Conference proceedings.) Yenimahalle, Ankara, Turkey: TMMOB/ATO.

Toke, D., & Nielsen, H. (2015). Policy consultation and political styles: Renewable energy consultations in the UK and Denmark. *British Politics*, *10*(4), 454–474.

Toonen, T. A. (1998). Networks, management and institutions: public administration as 'normal science'. *Public Administration*, *76*(2), 229–252.

Top, M., & Sungur, C. (2019). Opinions and evaluations of stakeholders in the implementation of the public-private partnership (PPP) model in integrated health campuses (city hospitals) in Turkey. *The International Journal of Health Planning and Management*, *34*(1), e241–e263.

Torfing, J. (2019). Collaborative innovation in the public sector: The argument. *Public Management Review*, *21*(1), 1–11.

Torfing, J., Sørensen, E., & Røiseland, A. (2019). Transforming the public sector into an arena for co-creation: Barriers, drivers, benefits, and ways forward. *Administration & Society*, *51*(5), 795–825.

Tsouros, A. (2009). City leadership for health and sustainable development: The World Health Organization European Healthy Cities Network. *Health Promotion International*, *24*(Suppl 1), i4–i10.

Turc, E., Guenoun, M., Rodrigues, M. Â. V., Demirkaya, Y., & Dupuis, J. (2016). Impacts of NPM-driven performance management reforms and ideologies in Napoleonic Local Governments: A comparative analysis of France, Portugal, and Turkey. In *Local Public Sector Reforms in Times of Crisis* (pp. 121–137). London: Palgrave Macmillan.

Üstüner, Y., & Yavuz, N. (2018). Turkey's Public Administration today: An overview and appraisal. *International Journal of Public Administration*, *41*(10), 820–831.

Van Ballaert, B. (2017). The European Commission's use of consultation during policy formulation: The effects of policy characteristics. *European Union Politics*, *18*(3), 406–423.

Van de Ven, A. H., & Ring, P. S. (2006). Relying on trust in cooperative inter-organizational relationships. *Handbook of Trust Research*, 144–164.

Van de Ven, A. H., & Walker, G. (1984). The dynamics of interorganizational coordination. *Administrative Science Quarterly*, 598–621.

Van Den Hooff, B., & De Ridder, J. A. (2004). Knowledge sharing in context: The influence of organizational commitment, communication climate and CMC use on knowledge sharing. *Journal of Knowledge Management*, *8*(6), 117–130.

Van Waarden, F. (1992). Dimensions and types of policy networks. *European Journal of Political Research*, *21*(1–2), 29–52.

Vujicic, M., Sparkes, S., & Mollahaliloğlu, S. (2009). *Health workforce policy in Turkey: Recent reforms and issues for the future*. Washington, DC: HNP World Bank.

Wartonick, B. D. (1986). Notes and Brief Reports. *Social Security Bulletin*, *49*(5), 21.

Wasserman, S., & Faust, K. (1994). *Social network analysis: Methods and applications* (Vol. 8). Cambridge: Cambridge University Press.

Wendt, C., Ağartan, T. I., & Kaminska, M. E. (2013). Social health insurance without corporate actors: Changes in self-regulation in Germany, Poland and Turkey. *Social Science & Medicine*, *86*, 88–95.

White, D., & Herzog, M. (2016). Examining state capacity in the context of electoral authoritarianism, regime formation and consolidation in Russia and Turkey. *Southeast European and Black Sea Studies*, *16*(4), 551–569.

Wilks, S. (2013). *The political power of the business corporation*. Nortampton, MA: Edward Elgar Publishing.

World Bank. (2010). World Bank Awards Turkey Health Transformation Program "Improving the lives of People in Europe and Central Asia" 2010 Competition. Retrieved from http://www.worldbank.org/en/news/press-release/2010/04/05/world-bank-awards-turkey-health-transformation-program-improving-the-lives-of-people-in-europe-and-central-asia-2010-competition

World Health Organization. (2012a). *Successful health system reforms: The case of Turkey*. Geneva: World Health Organization. Retrieved from https://dosyamerkez.saglik.gov.tr/Eklenti/2106,successful-health-system-reforms-the-case-of-turkeypdf.pdf?0

World Health Organization. (2012b). *Turkey health system performance assessment 2011*. A report by WHO Regional Office for Europe, Denmark, 3(10), 2017. Retrieved from http://www.euro.who.int/__data/assets/pdf_file/0004/165109/e95429.pdf

Yardım, M. S., Çilingiroğlu, N., & Yardım, N. (2013). Financial protection in health in Turkey: The effects of the Health Transformation Programme. *Health Policy and Planning*, *29*(2), 177–192.

Yıldız, M. (2007). E-government research: Reviewing the literature, limitations, and ways forward. *Government Information Quarterly*, *24*(3), 646–665.

Yıldız, M., & Babaoğlu, C. (2018). Public policy education in Turkey. In C. Bakır & G. Ertan (Eds.), *Policy analysis in Turkey* (pp. 271–288). Bristol: Bristol University Press.

Yilmaz, V. (2013). Changing origins of inequalities in access to health care services in Turkey: From occupational status to income. *New Perspectives on Turkey*, *48*, 55–77.

Yilmaz, F. O., Koç, E. M., Çil, V. D., & Kahveci, R. (2017). Evidence-based medicine and health technology assessments. *Family Practice and Palliative Care*, *2*(1), 17–22.

Zencirci, G. (2015a). Illusory debates: How the "Sadaka Culture" discourse masked the rise of social assistance in Turkey. *Asian Journal of Social Science*, *43*(1–2), 125–150.

Zencirci, G. (2015b). From property to civil society: The historical transformation of vakifs in modern Turkey (1923–2013). *International Journal of Middle East Studies*, *47*(3), 533–554.

Zheng, H., De Jong, M., & Koppenjan, J. (2010). Applying policy network theory to policy-making in China: The case of urban health insurance reform. *Public Administration*, *88*(2), 398–417.

Index

Note: Page numbers followed by "*n*" indicate footnotes.

Printed and bound by CPI Group (UK) Ltd, Croydon, CR0 4YY

13/09/2026

14961027-0008